The Connection Between Sleep and Health

Gabriella Goldberger

Published by Azure Time Press, 2023.

While every precaution has been taken in the preparation of this book, the publisher assumes no responsibility for errors or omissions, or for damages resulting from the use of the information contained herein.

THE CONNECTION BETWEEN SLEEP AND HEALTH

First edition. September 7, 2023.

ISBN: 979-8223794745

Written by Gabriella Goldberger.

Also by Gabriella Goldberger

Mindful Eating: Nourish Your Well-Being
Holistic Approaches to Stress Management
The Connection Between Sleep and Health

Table of Contents

To all those who have ever yearned for a peaceful night's sleep, and to those who tirelessly seek to understand the profound connection between sleep and health. May this book shed light on the mysteries of the night and guide you toward a future filled with restful slumber, vibrant days, and boundless well-being.

Chapter 1: Understanding Sleep

The Basics of Sleep: What Happens When You Sleep

When we lay our heads down each night and drift into slumber, our bodies embark on a remarkable journey through the world of sleep. It's a journey that is as mysterious as it is essential to our overall health and well-being.

As I begin this exploration, I can't help but marvel at the complexity and beauty of the human body's response to sleep. We all experience it, yet how often do we stop to ponder the intricate processes that unfold within us as we journey through the realms of dreams and rest?

Our journey starts with the very first moments of falling asleep. The transition from wakefulness to sleep isn't an abrupt one; instead, it's a gradual process guided by our internal body clock, known as the circadian rhythm. This rhythm influences when we feel alert and when we naturally start to wind down. It's an integral part of our sleep-wake cycle and plays a role in determining the quality of our sleep.

As we drift further into slumber, our brain activity undergoes a series of changes. We progress through various sleep stages, each with its unique characteristics. These stages are often divided into two broad categories: rapid eye movement (REM) sleep and non-REM (NREM) sleep. REM sleep is the stage where our most vivid dreams occur, and it's also when our brain activity resembles that of wakefulness. NREM sleep, on the other hand, is divided into three distinct stages, each with its own purpose in the restoration and maintenance of our physical and mental health.

One of the most crucial aspects of sleep is the opportunity it provides for our bodies to repair and rejuvenate. During the night, our cells go through a process of regeneration, and our immune system strengthens its defenses. It's no wonder that we often wake up feeling refreshed and energized after a good night's sleep; it's our body's way of saying, "Thank you for taking care of me."

But sleep isn't just a time for physical repair; it's also a time for mental processing and consolidation of memories. Our brains are incredibly active during REM sleep, sorting through the experiences of the day, and forming connections that help us learn and make sense of the world around us.

As we journey through the chapters of this book, we'll dive even deeper into the fascinating world of sleep. We'll explore the various sleep stages, discuss the factors that can disrupt our sleep patterns, and discover the profound impact that sleep has on our physical and mental health. So, join me as we continue our exploration, for there is much more to learn about the connection between sleep and our overall well-being.

The Sleep Cycle: Stages and Patterns

As we continue our journey into the world of sleep, it's crucial to explore the intricate dance of stages and patterns that make up the sleep cycle. Understanding the sleep cycle is like deciphering the rhythm of a beautifully composed symphony. Each stage has its unique role, and together, they orchestrate the harmonious restoration and rejuvenation of our bodies and minds.

Imagine this: you've closed your eyes, and you're drifting further into the realm of dreams. What happens next is a symphony of sleep, and it's a symphony composed of different movements, each with its own purpose.

Movement 1: NREM Sleep (Non-Rapid Eye Movement)

The sleep cycle begins with non-REM sleep, which is further divided into three stages: N1, N2, and N3. These stages are marked by distinct patterns of brain activity and physiological changes.

1. **Stage N1:** This is the lightest stage of non-REM sleep. During this phase, you may experience fleeting thoughts, and it's relatively easy to wake you up. Your muscles start to relax, and you might occasionally have muscle twitches.
2. **Stage N2:** As you progress to N2, your body temperature drops, and your heart rate becomes more regular. This is the stage where your

body prepares for deep sleep. Sleep spindles and K-complexes, two types of brain wave patterns, become prominent during this stage.

3. **Stage N3:** This is the deep sleep stage, also known as slow-wave sleep. During N3, your brain produces slow delta waves, and it's challenging to wake you up. This is when physical restoration primarily occurs, with growth hormone being released, muscles repaired, and energy restored.

Movement 2: REM Sleep (Rapid Eye Movement)

After the non-REM stages, we enter the fascinating world of REM sleep, which is characterized by rapid eye movements, increased brain activity, and vivid dreams. REM sleep is a vital part of the sleep cycle, playing a crucial role in cognitive functions, memory consolidation, and emotional well-being.

During REM sleep:

- Your brain is highly active, almost as active as when you're awake. This is when your most vivid and memorable dreams occur.
- Your eyes move rapidly beneath your closed eyelids, giving this stage its name.
- Your muscles become temporarily paralyzed to prevent you from physically acting out your dreams, a phenomenon known as REM atonia.

The sleep cycle isn't a one-time event that happens throughout the night; it's a repeating pattern. Typically, a complete sleep cycle takes about 90 to 110 minutes to cycle through all the stages, starting with non-REM sleep and progressing to REM sleep. Over the course of a night's sleep, you will go through multiple cycles, with each cycle providing essential benefits to your physical and mental well-being.

Now, you might be wondering, "How does my body decide which stage to enter next, and why do I sometimes wake up feeling groggy?" Well, the sleep cycle doesn't follow a rigid script; it's influenced by a variety of factors, including your circadian rhythm, sleep debt, and external environmental cues.

Your circadian rhythm, often referred to as your body's internal clock, plays a significant role in determining the timing and duration of your sleep cycles. It's why you naturally feel more awake and alert during the day and gradually become sleepier as the evening progresses.

Sleep debt, on the other hand, is accumulated when you don't get enough sleep over time. Your body tries to make up for this deficit during deep sleep stages (N3) by extending the duration of these stages. This is why it's crucial to prioritize consistent and adequate sleep to ensure you progress through the sleep cycles smoothly.

Environmental factors, such as noise, light, and temperature, can also influence the depth and quality of your sleep cycles. Creating a sleep-conducive environment that minimizes disturbances can significantly impact the effectiveness of your sleep cycles.

So, as we continue our exploration of sleep and its connection to health, remember that the sleep cycle is a symphony of stages and patterns, each contributing to your overall well-being. It's a dance that your body gracefully performs night after night, and understanding its rhythms can lead to improved sleep quality and a healthier, more energized you.

Circadian Rhythms: How Your Body's Internal Clock Works

Imagine your body as a finely tuned orchestra, and at the center of this orchestra is a conductor directing the performance. This conductor is none other than your body's internal clock, known as the circadian rhythm. Just like a conductor guides the musicians to create harmonious melodies, your circadian rhythm orchestrates your body's functions in a rhythmic and synchronized manner.

The Conductor of Your Body's Symphony: Circadian Rhythms

The term "circadian" comes from the Latin words "circa" (meaning "around") and "diem" (meaning "day"), which aptly describes the nature of these rhythms. Circadian rhythms are roughly 24-hour cycles that regulate various physiological processes, including sleep, wakefulness, body temperature, hormone release, and even mood. They ensure that our bodies are in sync with the natural day-night cycle of our environment.

Here's how the conductor, your circadian rhythm, directs the performance:

1. **The Sleep-Wake Cycle:** One of the most critical functions controlled by your circadian rhythm is the timing of your sleep and wakefulness. In the morning, as the sun rises and natural light increases, your circadian clock signals the release of cortisol, a hormone that helps you wake up and feel alert. Conversely, in the evening, as the sun sets and darkness falls, your body releases melatonin, a hormone that promotes sleepiness.

2. **Body Temperature:** Your body temperature is also subject to the guidance of your circadian rhythm. It typically starts to rise in the morning, helping you wake up, and reaches its peak in the late afternoon or early evening. As night falls, your body temperature begins to drop, which is conducive to falling asleep.

3. **Hormone Regulation:** Your circadian rhythm controls the release of various hormones, including cortisol, melatonin, growth hormone, and more. These hormones play essential roles in regulating metabolism, immune function, and tissue repair, all of which are closely tied to sleep and overall health.

4. **Mood and Alertness:** Disruptions to your circadian rhythm can have significant effects on mood and alertness. For example, shift workers or individuals with irregular sleep schedules may experience mood disturbances, increased stress, and reduced cognitive performance due to circadian misalignment.

Circadian Rhythm and the Modern Lifestyle

While our circadian rhythms are deeply ingrained in our biology, the demands of modern life can often challenge this natural rhythm. Late-night work, exposure to artificial light from screens, and travel across time zones can all disrupt our circadian rhythms.

The consequences of such disruptions can be profound. For instance, jet lag is a classic example of circadian misalignment when our internal clocks are out of sync with our new time zone. Symptoms include fatigue, insomnia, and reduced cognitive performance. Similarly, shift work, which requires individuals to be awake and alert during nighttime hours, can lead to circadian disruptions and long-term health issues.

Understanding your circadian rhythm and respecting its natural ebb and flow can help you maintain a healthy sleep-wake cycle. Here are some tips to stay in harmony with your internal clock:

1. **Maintain a Consistent Schedule:** Try to wake up and go to bed at the same times every day, even on weekends. Consistency reinforces your circadian rhythm.
2. **Exposure to Natural Light:** Spend time outdoors during the day, especially in the morning. Natural light helps regulate your internal clock and promotes alertness.
3. **Limit Artificial Light at Night:** In the evening, reduce exposure to screens and artificial lighting, especially in the hour or two before bedtime. The blue light emitted by screens can interfere with melatonin production and delay sleep.
4. **Be Mindful of Meals:** Eating large or heavy meals close to bedtime can disrupt your sleep. Aim to have your last meal at least a few hours before bedtime.
5. **Travel with Care:** If you're crossing time zones, adjust your schedule gradually to align with your destination's time zone before you travel.

By acknowledging the conductor within you, your circadian rhythm, and taking steps to support its natural rhythm, you can improve your sleep quality and overall well-being. In the grand symphony of your life, a well-tuned circadian rhythm ensures that each note is played in harmony, creating a healthier, more energized you.

Sleep Duration: How Much Sleep Do You Really Need?

In our fast-paced, 24/7 world, where productivity and constant connectivity often take precedence, it's easy to overlook one fundamental aspect of our lives: sleep duration. How much sleep do we truly need to function optimally and maintain our overall well-being?

The Sleep Duration Spectrum

Sleep duration isn't a one-size-fits-all equation. Just as we have individual tastes, preferences, and unique physical characteristics, our sleep needs can also vary. The optimal amount of sleep differs from person to person, and it can change over the course of our lives.

Let's explore the sleep duration spectrum:

1. **Short Sleepers:** Some individuals naturally require less sleep than others. They thrive on just a few hours of sleep each night without experiencing significant negative effects. However, true short sleepers are rare, and most people who believe they fall into this category may, in fact, be suffering from chronic sleep deprivation.
2. **Average Sleepers:** The majority of adults require between 7 to 9 hours of sleep per night to function optimally. Within this range, there's room for variability, and some people may feel their best with 7 hours while others need a full 9 hours.
3. **Long Sleepers:** On the opposite end of the spectrum, some individuals require more sleep than the average range to feel rested and alert. Long sleepers may need up to 10 or even 11 hours of sleep per night.

The Myth of the 8-Hour Rule

You've likely heard the common advice that adults need 8 hours of sleep per night. While this is a useful guideline, it doesn't account for individual variability. In reality, the optimal sleep duration depends on various factors, including age, genetics, lifestyle, and overall health.

Factors influencing your ideal sleep duration:

- **Age:** Sleep needs change throughout the lifespan. Infants and teenagers typically need more sleep, while older adults may require less.
- **Genetics:** Some genetic variations can influence your sleep patterns and how much sleep you naturally need.
- **Lifestyle:** Your daily activities, stress levels, and physical demands can impact your sleep requirements.
- **Health:** Certain medical conditions or medications may affect your sleep needs.
- **Quality of Sleep:** The quality of your sleep matters as much as the quantity. Restorative sleep in fewer hours can be more beneficial than longer, disrupted sleep.

Listen to Your Body

The best way to determine your ideal sleep duration is to listen to your body. Pay attention to how you feel during the day. Do you feel alert and focused, or are you constantly battling fatigue and brain fog?

Here are some signs that you may not be getting enough sleep:

- **Daytime Sleepiness:** Feeling excessively tired during the day, especially after lunch, is a red flag for inadequate sleep.
- **Irritability and Mood Swings:** Lack of sleep can lead to mood disturbances, making you more irritable, anxious, or depressed.
- **Difficulty Concentrating:** If you find it challenging to stay focused and productive, it may be due to insufficient sleep.
- **Frequent Illness:** A weakened immune system can result from chronic sleep deprivation, making you more susceptible to illnesses.
- **Weight Gain:** Poor sleep can disrupt the balance of hunger-regulating hormones, leading to weight gain.

Finding Your Sleep Sweet Spot

To identify your optimal sleep duration, start by giving yourself the opportunity to sleep without an alarm clock when you have a few consecutive days off. Allow your body to naturally wake up, and note the number of hours you've slept. This can serve as a baseline to gauge how much sleep you truly need.

Once you have a better understanding of your sleep needs, strive to create a sleep schedule that accommodates your ideal sleep duration. Prioritize sleep as an essential component of your daily routine, just like eating a balanced diet and staying physically active.

In summary, sleep duration is not a fixed number but a personal range influenced by numerous factors. The key is to find your individual sleep sweet spot, where you wake up feeling refreshed, alert, and ready to tackle the day. By prioritizing your sleep needs and allowing your body to dictate its own sleep duration, you can optimize your overall well-being and thrive in all aspects of life.

Factors Affecting Sleep: Genetics, Age, and Lifestyle

As we continue our journey into the realm of sleep, we'll explore the intricate web of factors that influence the quality and quantity of our slumber. Sleep is a deeply personal experience, shaped by a combination of genetics, age, and lifestyle choices.

Genetics: The Sleep Blueprint

Much of our sleep architecture is determined by our genetic makeup. Genes play a significant role in shaping our circadian rhythms, sleep cycles, and even our vulnerability to sleep disorders. Think of your genes as the blueprint for your sleep patterns.

1. **Circadian Rhythms:** Genetic variations can influence your natural sleep-wake timing. Some people are "morning people," with a genetic predisposition to be most alert and energetic in the early hours, while others are "night owls," feeling more active and awake during the evening.

2. **Sleep Duration:** Genetic factors also contribute to how much sleep you naturally require. As mentioned earlier, short sleepers and long sleepers often have genetic underpinnings that determine their sleep duration needs.

3. **Sleep Disorders:** Certain sleep disorders, such as narcolepsy and restless legs syndrome, can have a hereditary component. If these conditions run in your family, you may be at a higher risk of developing them.

While genetics can set the stage for your sleep patterns, it's essential to remember that lifestyle choices and environmental factors can significantly modulate these genetic predispositions.

Age: Sleep Through the Lifespan

Sleep is not a static phenomenon; it evolves over the course of our lives. Understanding how sleep changes with age is crucial to maintaining healthy sleep patterns.

1. **Infants and Children:** Babies spend a significant portion of their early lives sleeping, with sleep gradually consolidating into more extended nighttime periods. Adolescents often experience a shift in their circadian rhythms, leading to later bedtimes and waking times.

2. **Adults:** In early adulthood, most people require 7 to 9 hours of sleep per night. However, sleep quality and sleep disorders can begin to affect sleep patterns. As adults age, they may experience more fragmented sleep and earlier wake times.

3. **Older Adults:** Seniors often experience changes in sleep architecture, including a decrease in deep sleep (N3) and an increase in light sleep and awakenings. These changes can result in more frequent awakenings during the night and a tendency to wake up earlier in the morning.

Lifestyle Choices: Nurturing or Disrupting Sleep

Our daily choices and habits play a significant role in shaping our sleep quality. The lifestyle factors that can either nurture or disrupt our sleep include:

1. **Diet:** Consuming caffeine, alcohol, or heavy meals close to bedtime can interfere with sleep. Opt for lighter evening meals and avoid stimulants in the hours leading up to sleep.

2. **Physical Activity:** Regular exercise can improve sleep quality, but intense workouts close to bedtime can have the opposite effect. Aim for moderate exercise earlier in the day.

3. **Stress and Mental Health:** Chronic stress, anxiety, and mood disorders can disrupt sleep. Practices like meditation and relaxation techniques can help manage stress and improve sleep.

4. **Screen Time:** Exposure to the blue light emitted by screens before bedtime can interfere with the production of melatonin, a hormone that promotes sleep. Create a technology-free bedtime routine to prepare your body for rest.

5. **Sleep Environment:** Factors like noise, light, and room temperature can impact sleep quality. Creating a sleep-conducive environment with blackout curtains, white noise machines, and comfortable bedding can enhance your sleep experience.

6. **Work and Social Commitments:** Irregular work hours, frequent travel, and social obligations can disrupt sleep schedules. Strive for a consistent sleep routine, even on weekends.

Balancing the Equation: Genetics, Age, and Lifestyle

Optimal sleep is a delicate balance between our genetic predispositions, the changing needs of our bodies as we age, and the daily choices we make. To achieve a harmonious relationship with sleep, consider these key principles:

1. **Know Your Sleep Needs:** Understand your genetic tendencies and how they interact with your age-related sleep changes. Tailor your sleep routine accordingly.

2. **Prioritize Sleep Hygiene:** Make healthy sleep habits a daily practice by creating a sleep-conducive environment and following a consistent

sleep schedule.

3. **Adapt and Adjust:** Be flexible in adapting your sleep routine to life changes while respecting the core principles of good sleep hygiene.

By recognizing the role of genetics, age, and lifestyle in your sleep patterns, you can take proactive steps to nurture healthy sleep and, in turn, enhance your overall well-being. Sleep becomes not just a passive state, but an active choice in crafting a fulfilling life.

Chapter 2: Sleep and Physical Health

Sleep and the Immune System: How Sleep Boosts Your Body's Defenses

In the intricate dance between sleep and physical health, one of the most compelling and vital partnerships is that between sleep and the immune system. Your immune system is your body's primary defense mechanism against infections, and it relies on a well-rested body to function optimally.

The Immune System: Your Inner Shield

Before we dive into the relationship between sleep and the immune system, let's take a moment to appreciate the complexity of this remarkable defense network within your body. Your immune system is a sophisticated army of cells, proteins, and tissues that work tirelessly to protect you from harmful invaders like viruses, bacteria, and even cancer cells.

Two primary branches of the immune system are innate immunity and adaptive immunity. Innate immunity provides immediate but general defense against pathogens, while adaptive immunity develops over time, providing targeted and long-lasting protection. Both branches depend on the quality and effectiveness of your immune responses, which are significantly influenced by your sleep patterns.

Sleep: A Natural Immune Booster

It turns out that sleep is one of your body's most potent weapons when it comes to strengthening your immune system. Here's how it works:

1. **Cytokine Production:** While you sleep, your body produces a variety of immune-boosting substances, such as cytokines. These proteins play a crucial role in cell signaling and help coordinate the immune response to infections and inflammation. Inadequate sleep can lead to reduced cytokine production, impairing your body's ability to combat pathogens effectively.
2. **Immune Cell Activity:** Your immune system deploys specialized

cells, like T cells and natural killer (NK) cells, to identify and destroy infected or abnormal cells. These cells are more active during deep sleep, particularly in the stage known as slow-wave sleep (N3). Insufficient sleep can hinder their effectiveness, leaving you more vulnerable to infections.

3. **Antibody Production:** During REM sleep, your body produces antibodies, which are proteins that target specific pathogens. Adequate REM sleep is essential for the creation of a robust immune response. If you're not getting enough REM sleep, your body may struggle to develop the necessary defenses against infectious agents.

4. **Inflammation Regulation:** Sleep helps regulate the balance of pro-inflammatory and anti-inflammatory cytokines. Chronic sleep deprivation can lead to an overproduction of pro-inflammatory cytokines, contributing to inflammation-related health issues like heart disease, diabetes, and autoimmune disorders.

The Consequences of Sleep Deprivation

When you consistently fail to get enough sleep, your immune system pays a steep price. Here are some of the consequences of chronic sleep deprivation on your immune health:

1. **Increased Susceptibility:** Sleep-deprived individuals are more susceptible to infections, including the common cold and flu. Their immune systems struggle to mount a robust defense, making them easy targets for invading pathogens.

2. **Slower Recovery:** When you do get sick, recovery can be slower and more challenging if you're not well-rested. Sleep is a vital part of the healing process, as it supports the immune response and helps repair damaged tissues.

3. **Vaccination Effectiveness:** Sleep deprivation can reduce the effectiveness of vaccines. Adequate sleep before and after vaccination is crucial to ensure your body produces a strong immune response.

4. **Chronic Health Conditions:** Long-term sleep deprivation is associated with an increased risk of chronic health conditions,

including cardiovascular disease, diabetes, and autoimmune disorders. These conditions are often linked to immune dysfunction.

Prioritizing Sleep for Immune Health

It's clear that sleep is a powerful ally in maintaining a robust immune system. To bolster your immune health through sleep, consider these strategies:

1. **Establish a Consistent Sleep Schedule:** Go to bed and wake up at the same times every day to reinforce your body's circadian rhythm.
2. **Create a Sleep-Conducive Environment:** Make your bedroom comfortable, dark, and quiet. Ensure your mattress and pillows provide adequate support.
3. **Limit Screen Time Before Bed:** Avoid screens for at least an hour before bedtime to minimize exposure to blue light, which can disrupt sleep.
4. **Manage Stress:** Practice stress-reduction techniques like meditation, deep breathing, or yoga to calm your mind before sleep.
5. **Limit Caffeine and Alcohol:** Both substances can interfere with sleep quality, so use them in moderation and avoid them close to bedtime.
6. **Prioritize Sleep Hygiene:** Develop a bedtime routine that signals to your body that it's time to wind down and prepare for sleep.

In the intricate relationship between sleep and your immune system, prioritizing healthy sleep habits becomes a powerful strategy for protecting your body from infections and promoting overall well-being. By understanding the vital role of sleep in immune function, you can nurture this symbiotic relationship and strengthen your inner shield against illness.

The Role of Sleep in Weight Management and Metabolism

As we delve deeper into the multifaceted connection between sleep and physical health, it's crucial to recognize the significant role that sleep plays in weight management and metabolism. Sleep isn't just a passive state; it actively influences how your body processes and stores energy.

Metabolism: The Body's Energy Regulator

Before we dive into the relationship between sleep and metabolism, let's clarify what metabolism means. Metabolism encompasses all the biochemical processes in your body that convert food into energy and maintain your bodily functions. It's the engine that keeps you running.

Two key components of metabolism are:

1. **Basal Metabolic Rate (BMR):** This represents the energy your body expends at rest to maintain basic functions like breathing, circulation, and cell production.
2. **Energy Expenditure:** This includes the calories you burn through physical activity and digestion.

Your metabolism can be influenced by various factors, including genetics, age, muscle mass, and, as we'll explore in detail, sleep patterns.

Sleep and Your Metabolism

Sleep and metabolism share a complex and bidirectional relationship. Here's how sleep influences your metabolic processes:

1. **Hormonal Regulation:** Sleep plays a vital role in regulating hormones that affect hunger and appetite. Ghrelin, a hormone that stimulates hunger, increases with sleep deprivation, leading to greater food intake. Conversely, leptin, a hormone that signals fullness, decreases with insufficient sleep, contributing to overeating.
2. **Insulin Sensitivity:** Chronic sleep deprivation can lead to reduced insulin sensitivity, similar to the effects of insulin resistance. This can increase the risk of type 2 diabetes and weight gain.
3. **Cortisol Levels:** Sleep deprivation can elevate cortisol levels, a stress hormone that can promote fat storage, particularly around the abdominal area.
4. **Increased Caloric Intake:** Sleep-deprived individuals often consume more calories, especially from high-fat and high-carbohydrate foods, as they seek quick sources of energy to combat fatigue.

5. **Energy Balance:** Poor sleep can disrupt the balance between energy intake (calories consumed) and energy expenditure (calories burned). This imbalance can lead to weight gain over time.

The Consequences of Sleep Deprivation on Weight and Health

The consequences of chronic sleep deprivation on weight and health are far-reaching:

1. **Weight Gain:** Sleep deprivation is associated with weight gain and obesity. Even modest sleep restrictions can lead to an increase in body weight.
2. **Increased Risk of Obesity-Related Diseases:** Poor sleep quality and duration are linked to an increased risk of obesity-related conditions such as type 2 diabetes, cardiovascular disease, and hypertension.
3. **Disrupted Appetite Regulation:** Insufficient sleep can disrupt the hormones that regulate appetite, leading to overeating and unhealthy food choices.
4. **Muscle Mass Loss:** Sleep deprivation can cause the loss of lean muscle mass, reducing your body's ability to burn calories efficiently.
5. **Mental Health Impact:** Sleep deprivation can affect mood and mental health, potentially leading to emotional eating and weight gain.

Prioritizing Sleep for Weight Management and Metabolism

If you're looking to support your weight management and overall health, improving your sleep habits is a vital step. Here are some strategies to optimize your sleep for metabolism:

1. **Consistent Sleep Schedule:** Go to bed and wake up at the same times each day, even on weekends, to reinforce your body's internal clock.
2. **Create a Sleep-Conducive Environment:** Make your bedroom dark, quiet, and comfortable for restful sleep.
3. **Limit Screen Time:** Avoid screens for at least an hour before

      bedtime to minimize exposure to blue light.

4. **Control Stress:** Practice stress-reduction techniques like meditation, deep breathing, or progressive muscle relaxation to relax your mind and body before sleep.
5. **Moderate Caffeine and Alcohol:** Limit the consumption of caffeine and alcohol, especially close to bedtime.
6. **Prioritize Sleep Hygiene:** Establish a bedtime routine that signals to your body that it's time to wind down and prepare for sleep.

In the intricate dance between sleep and metabolism, nurturing healthy sleep habits becomes a powerful strategy for supporting weight management and overall well-being. By recognizing the profound impact of sleep on your metabolic processes, you can harness the potential for a healthier body and a more balanced life.

Sleep and Cardiovascular Health: Impact on Heart and Blood Pressure

In our exploration of the intricate relationship between sleep and physical health, we turn our attention to the vital connection between sleep and cardiovascular health. Your heart is a tireless worker, pumping blood throughout your body day and night. Sleep plays a profound role in maintaining the health of your cardiovascular system, affecting heart function, blood pressure regulation, and the risk of heart disease.

The Heart's Nightly Symphony

Your heart doesn't rest when you doze off; in fact, it maintains a steady rhythm during sleep that is finely tuned to the stages of your sleep cycle. This rhythmic pattern is orchestrated by your body's internal clock, your circadian rhythm, and it's essential for cardiovascular health.

Here's how sleep affects your heart and blood pressure:

1. **Blood Pressure Regulation:** During deep sleep stages, such as slow-wave sleep (N3), your blood pressure naturally decreases. This drop in blood pressure allows your cardiovascular system to relax and recover from the demands of the day. Chronic sleep deprivation can disrupt

this natural decline, leading to sustained high blood pressure.

2. **Heart Rate Variability:** A healthy heart doesn't beat like a metronome; it exhibits variability in the time intervals between heartbeats. This variability is a sign of a robust and adaptable cardiovascular system. Quality sleep, especially during REM sleep, is associated with improved heart rate variability.

3. **Inflammation Control:** Poor sleep quality and insufficient sleep can lead to increased levels of inflammation in the body, including the cardiovascular system. Chronic inflammation is a risk factor for heart disease.

4. **Cardiac Events:** Sleep plays a role in triggering cardiac events. Research shows that heart attacks and sudden cardiac deaths are more likely to occur in the early morning hours, often following disrupted or inadequate sleep.

The Consequences of Sleep Deprivation on Cardiovascular Health

Chronic sleep deprivation can have profound and far-reaching consequences for your cardiovascular health:

1. **Hypertension:** Long-term sleep deprivation can lead to high blood pressure, a significant risk factor for heart disease, stroke, and other cardiovascular conditions.

2. **Heart Disease:** Insufficient sleep is associated with an increased risk of developing heart disease. It can contribute to the accumulation of plaque in the arteries (atherosclerosis) and raise the risk of heart attacks and strokes.

3. **Arrhythmias:** Sleep disturbances, such as sleep apnea, can disrupt the heart's electrical activity and lead to arrhythmias, irregular heartbeats that can have serious health implications.

4. **Heart Failure:** Chronic sleep deprivation can strain the heart and contribute to the development or worsening of heart failure.

Prioritizing Sleep for Cardiovascular Health

To support your cardiovascular health, it's essential to prioritize healthy sleep habits. Here are some strategies to optimize your sleep for the sake of your heart:

1. **Maintain a Consistent Sleep Schedule:** Go to bed and wake up at the same times every day to reinforce your body's circadian rhythm.
2. **Create a Relaxing Sleep Environment:** Make your bedroom conducive to rest by keeping it dark, quiet, and cool.
3. **Limit Screen Time:** Avoid screens for at least an hour before bedtime to minimize exposure to stimulating blue light.
4. **Manage Stress:** Practice relaxation techniques such as meditation, deep breathing, or progressive muscle relaxation to reduce stress levels, which can contribute to sleep disturbances.
5. **Moderate Caffeine and Alcohol:** Limit the consumption of caffeine and alcohol, especially close to bedtime.
6. **Prioritize Sleep Hygiene:** Establish a bedtime routine that signals to your body that it's time to wind down and prepare for sleep.

By recognizing the profound impact of sleep on your cardiovascular health, you can take proactive steps to protect your heart and reduce the risk of heart disease. A healthy heart is a priceless asset, and quality sleep is a fundamental building block in maintaining its well-being.

Hormones and Sleep: The Connection Between Sleep and Hormonal Balance

In our ongoing exploration of the intricate relationship between sleep and physical health, we now turn our attention to the profound impact that sleep has on your hormonal balance. Hormones act as messengers within your body, regulating essential functions like growth, metabolism, mood, and more. Sleep plays a pivotal role in maintaining the delicate equilibrium of these hormonal systems.

The Hormonal Symphony of Sleep

Imagine your body as a complex orchestra of hormones, each playing a unique instrument in harmony to create the symphony of your daily life. While this orchestra operates around the clock, it has a particular tempo and rhythm that is orchestrated by your sleep-wake cycle.

Here's how sleep influences your hormonal balance:

1. **Growth Hormone:** One of the most critical hormones affected by sleep is growth hormone. It's during deep sleep, particularly in the slow-wave sleep stage (N3), that your body releases the highest levels of growth hormone. This hormone is essential for tissue repair, muscle growth, and overall physical well-being.
2. **Cortisol:** Cortisol is a hormone produced by your adrenal glands in response to stress and low blood glucose levels. Normally, cortisol levels follow a diurnal pattern, peaking in the morning to help you wake up and gradually declining throughout the day. However, chronic sleep deprivation can lead to elevated cortisol levels at night, disrupting this natural rhythm and increasing stress.
3. **Melatonin:** The hormone melatonin is often associated with sleep, but it's also a key player in regulating your circadian rhythm. Exposure to light, especially blue light from screens, can suppress melatonin production, making it harder to fall asleep and disrupting your internal clock.
4. **Leptin and Ghrelin:** These hormones are involved in appetite regulation. Leptin signals fullness and reduces appetite, while ghrelin stimulates hunger. Sleep deprivation can disrupt the balance of these hormones, leading to increased appetite and overeating.
5. **Insulin:** Sleep plays a significant role in regulating blood sugar levels and insulin sensitivity. Chronic sleep deprivation can lead to insulin resistance, increasing the risk of type 2 diabetes.

The Consequences of Sleep Disruptions on Hormonal Health

Disruptions in your sleep patterns, whether they stem from sleep disorders, poor sleep quality, or irregular sleep schedules, can have profound consequences for your hormonal health:

1. **Weight Gain:** Sleep disruptions can lead to imbalances in leptin and

ghrelin, increasing appetite and promoting weight gain.

2. **Metabolic Disorders:** Chronic sleep deprivation is associated with insulin resistance, contributing to the development of metabolic disorders like type 2 diabetes.

3. **Stress and Anxiety:** Elevated cortisol levels due to sleep disturbances can lead to increased stress, anxiety, and mood disorders.

4. **Hormonal Imbalance:** Irregular sleep patterns can disrupt the release of hormones like growth hormone and melatonin, potentially impacting overall health and well-being.

Prioritizing Sleep for Hormonal Balance

To support hormonal balance and overall health, it's essential to prioritize healthy sleep habits. Here are some strategies to optimize your sleep for hormonal well-being:

1. **Establish a Consistent Sleep Schedule:** Go to bed and wake up at the same times every day to reinforce your body's circadian rhythm.

2. **Create a Sleep-Conducive Environment:** Make your bedroom dark, quiet, and comfortable for restful sleep.

3. **Limit Screen Time:** Avoid screens for at least an hour before bedtime to minimize exposure to stimulating blue light.

4. **Manage Stress:** Practice relaxation techniques such as meditation, deep breathing, or progressive muscle relaxation to reduce stress levels.

5. **Moderate Caffeine and Alcohol:** Limit the consumption of caffeine and alcohol, especially close to bedtime.

6. **Prioritize Sleep Hygiene:** Establish a bedtime routine that signals to your body that it's time to wind down and prepare for sleep.

By recognizing the profound impact of sleep on your hormonal balance, you can take proactive steps to nurture your overall well-being. A harmonious hormonal orchestra, conducted by healthy sleep habits, ensures that your body functions optimally and that you thrive in all aspects of life.

How Sleep Affects Pain Perception and Chronic Conditions

In our exploration of the intricate relationship between sleep and physical health, we now turn our focus to the profound impact of sleep on pain perception and chronic health conditions. Sleep is not just a passive state; it actively influences your body's ability to manage pain and cope with chronic illnesses.

Sleep and Pain Perception: The Pain-Sleep Cycle

Pain and sleep share a complex and bidirectional relationship. When you experience pain, it can disrupt your sleep, and conversely, poor sleep can heighten your sensitivity to pain. This intricate interplay can have significant implications for your overall well-being.

Here's how sleep affects pain perception:

1. **Pain Modulation:** During deep sleep stages, such as slow-wave sleep (N3), your body's pain modulation system is particularly active. This means that deep sleep can help reduce pain perception and enhance your ability to cope with discomfort.
2. **Endogenous Pain Control:** Sleep supports the release of endogenous pain control mechanisms, such as the body's natural pain-relieving chemicals like endorphins and enkephalins. Insufficient sleep can hinder the effectiveness of these mechanisms.
3. **Sensory Thresholds:** Sleep deprivation can lower your pain thresholds, making you more sensitive to pain. What might be a mild discomfort during restorative sleep can become excruciating when you're sleep-deprived.
4. **Emotional Impact:** Poor sleep can exacerbate the emotional toll of pain. Sleep disruptions are associated with increased anxiety, depression, and irritability, all of which can intensify the perception of pain.

Chronic Conditions and Sleep: A Vicious Cycle

Chronic health conditions often coexist with sleep disturbances, creating a challenging cycle that can be difficult to break. Some chronic conditions that are influenced by sleep include:

1. **Chronic Pain:** Conditions like fibromyalgia, arthritis, and chronic migraines are often accompanied by sleep disturbances. The pain itself can disrupt sleep, leading to fatigue and increased pain sensitivity.
2. **Mental Health Disorders:** Conditions like depression, anxiety, and post-traumatic stress disorder can lead to sleep disturbances, and poor sleep can exacerbate the symptoms of these disorders.
3. **Neurological Disorders:** Conditions such as Parkinson's disease and restless legs syndrome can disrupt sleep, leading to daytime fatigue and worsening motor symptoms.
4. **Cardiovascular Conditions:** Sleep apnea, a common sleep disorder, is associated with an increased risk of heart disease, hypertension, and stroke.
5. **Metabolic Disorders:** Sleep disturbances are linked to metabolic conditions like obesity and type 2 diabetes, and they can contribute to the progression of these diseases.

The Consequences of Sleep Disruptions on Pain and Chronic Conditions

Sleep disruptions can intensify the experience of pain and exacerbate the symptoms of chronic conditions in several ways:

1. **Increased Pain Perception:** Poor sleep can heighten your sensitivity to pain, making chronic pain conditions more difficult to manage.
2. **Reduced Pain Tolerance:** Sleep deprivation can lower your pain threshold, meaning you may experience pain more intensely than you would with adequate sleep.
3. **Inflammation:** Chronic sleep disturbances can contribute to systemic inflammation, which can worsen the symptoms of many chronic conditions.
4. **Mood and Cognitive Function:** Sleep disruptions can lead to mood

disturbances and cognitive impairment, making it more challenging to manage chronic health conditions effectively.

Prioritizing Sleep for Pain Management and Chronic Conditions

If you're dealing with pain or a chronic health condition, optimizing your sleep is essential for symptom management and overall well-being. Here are some strategies to improve your sleep quality:

1. **Establish a Consistent Sleep Schedule:** Go to bed and wake up at the same times every day to reinforce your body's circadian rhythm.
2. **Create a Sleep-Conducive Environment:** Make your bedroom dark, quiet, and comfortable for restful sleep.
3. **Limit Screen Time:** Avoid screens for at least an hour before bedtime to minimize exposure to stimulating blue light.
4. **Manage Stress:** Practice relaxation techniques such as meditation, deep breathing, or progressive muscle relaxation to reduce stress levels.
5. **Moderate Caffeine and Alcohol:** Limit the consumption of caffeine and alcohol, especially close to bedtime.
6. **Prioritize Sleep Hygiene:** Establish a bedtime routine that signals to your body that it's time to wind down and prepare for sleep.

By recognizing the profound impact of sleep on pain perception and chronic conditions, you can take proactive steps to improve your overall well-being. Quality sleep becomes not just a passive state, but a powerful tool for managing pain and promoting a healthier life, even in the face of chronic health challenges.

Chapter 3: Sleep and Mental Health

Sleep and Emotional Regulation: How It Influences Mood

In our exploration of the vital connection between sleep and mental health, we now venture into the fascinating realm of emotional regulation. Sleep is a linchpin in maintaining emotional well-being, as it directly influences mood, stress levels, and your ability to navigate the complex terrain of your emotions.

Sleep and the Emotional Rollercoaster

Emotions are an integral part of the human experience, shaping our perceptions, interactions, and overall quality of life. The way we perceive, process, and manage emotions is closely tied to the quality and quantity of our sleep.

Here's how sleep influences emotional regulation:

1. **Emotion Processing:** During sleep, particularly in the rapid eye movement (REM) stage, your brain processes and consolidates emotional experiences from the day. This helps you make sense of emotions, reduce their intensity, and integrate them into your emotional well-being.
2. **Stress Response:** Sleep plays a pivotal role in regulating the body's stress response. Adequate sleep helps you manage stress more effectively, while sleep deprivation can lead to heightened stress levels and emotional reactivity.
3. **Emotional Resilience:** Good sleep enhances your emotional resilience, helping you cope with life's challenges and bounce back from emotional setbacks.
4. **Negative Bias:** Sleep disruptions can tilt your emotional responses toward negativity, making you more prone to pessimism, irritability, and emotional overreactions.
5. **Impaired Emotional Regulation:** Chronic sleep deprivation can impair your ability to regulate emotions, leading to mood disorders like anxiety and depression.

The Consequences of Sleep Disruptions on Mood and Mental Health

The impact of sleep disruptions on mood and mental health is profound and multifaceted:

1. **Mood Disorders:** Sleep disturbances are closely linked to mood disorders such as depression and anxiety. Chronic sleep deprivation can exacerbate these conditions and make them more challenging to manage.
2. **Emotional Reactivity:** Sleep-deprived individuals are more likely to experience intense emotional reactions and have difficulty controlling their responses to emotional stimuli.
3. **Impaired Decision-Making:** Poor sleep can impair your judgment and decision-making abilities, leading to emotional distress and regrets.
4. **Reduced Resilience:** Sleep disruptions can reduce your capacity to cope with life's challenges, making you more vulnerable to emotional breakdowns.
5. **Interpersonal Relationships:** Sleep-deprived individuals often struggle with irritability and conflicts in their relationships, which can further contribute to mood disturbances.

Prioritizing Sleep for Emotional Regulation and Mental Health

To support your emotional regulation and overall mental health, it's crucial to prioritize healthy sleep habits. Here are some strategies to optimize your sleep for emotional well-being:

1. **Establish a Consistent Sleep Schedule:** Go to bed and wake up at the same times every day to reinforce your body's circadian rhythm.
2. **Create a Sleep-Conducive Environment:** Make your bedroom dark, quiet, and comfortable for restful sleep.
3. **Limit Screen Time:** Avoid screens for at least an hour before bedtime to minimize exposure to stimulating blue light.
4. **Manage Stress:** Practice relaxation techniques such as meditation, deep breathing, or progressive muscle relaxation to reduce stress

levels.

5. **Moderate Caffeine and Alcohol:** Limit the consumption of caffeine and alcohol, especially close to bedtime.
6. **Prioritize Sleep Hygiene:** Establish a bedtime routine that signals to your body that it's time to wind down and prepare for sleep.

By recognizing the profound impact of sleep on emotional regulation and mental health, you can take proactive steps to improve your overall well-being. Quality sleep becomes a powerful ally in navigating the complex landscape of emotions, fostering resilience, and promoting a happier, more balanced life.

Sleep and Stress: The Bidirectional Relationship

In our exploration of the intricate relationship between sleep and mental health, we now delve into the dynamic interplay between sleep and stress. Stress is an inherent part of life, and how you sleep can significantly impact how you experience and manage stress. Likewise, stress can disrupt your sleep patterns.

The Dance of Sleep and Stress

Sleep and stress are like dance partners, each influencing the other in a continuous rhythmic pattern. Understanding this dynamic relationship is essential for managing both stress and sleep effectively.

Here's how sleep influences stress and vice versa:

1. **Stress and Sleep Quality:** When you're stressed, your body's stress response, driven by the release of hormones like cortisol, can disrupt your sleep patterns. Stress-induced hyperarousal can make it challenging to fall asleep, stay asleep, or experience restorative sleep.
2. **Sleep and Stress Resilience:** Quality sleep is crucial for building emotional resilience and the ability to cope with stress. When you're well-rested, you're better equipped to handle life's challenges and bounce back from stressors.
3. **Emotional Regulation:** Sleep plays a pivotal role in regulating emotions. Inadequate sleep can lead to increased emotional reactivity, making you more susceptible to stress-induced mood disturbances.

4. **Cognitive Function:** Sleep is essential for clear thinking and problem-solving. Sleep-deprived individuals may find it harder to manage stress and make sound decisions.

5. **Stress-Related Sleep Disorders:** Chronic stress can lead to the development of sleep disorders like insomnia and hypersomnia (excessive sleepiness), further exacerbating sleep disturbances.

The Consequences of Chronic Stress on Sleep and Mental Health

Chronic stress can have far-reaching consequences on both sleep and mental health:

1. **Insomnia:** Persistent stress can lead to insomnia, characterized by difficulty falling asleep, staying asleep, or waking up too early. This can create a vicious cycle, as poor sleep further amplifies stress levels.

2. **Hypersomnia:** In some cases, chronic stress can trigger excessive sleepiness, causing individuals to sleep excessively. This can be a sign of depression or other mood disorders.

3. **Mood Disorders:** Chronic stress is a significant risk factor for mood disorders such as anxiety and depression. These conditions often coexist with sleep disturbances.

4. **Cognitive Impairment:** Prolonged stress can impair cognitive function, leading to difficulties in concentration, memory, and problem-solving.

5. **Physical Health Implications:** Chronic stress is associated with an increased risk of physical health problems, including cardiovascular disease, digestive disorders, and immune system dysfunction.

Strategies to Foster a Harmonious Relationship

To foster a harmonious relationship between sleep and stress, consider implementing the following strategies:

1. **Stress Management:** Develop effective stress management techniques, such as mindfulness meditation, deep breathing exercises, or yoga, to reduce stress levels.

2. **Establish a Sleep Routine:** Create a consistent sleep schedule and bedtime routine to signal to your body that it's time to wind down and prepare for rest.
3. **Limit Screen Time:** Avoid screens for at least an hour before bedtime to minimize exposure to stimulating blue light.
4. **Physical Activity:** Engage in regular physical activity, but avoid intense workouts close to bedtime, as they can be stimulating.
5. **Nutrition:** Maintain a balanced diet and avoid heavy or spicy meals close to bedtime. Limit caffeine and alcohol intake, especially in the evening.
6. **Sleep Hygiene:** Create a comfortable sleep environment by keeping your bedroom dark, quiet, and at a comfortable temperature.

By recognizing the bidirectional relationship between sleep and stress, you can take proactive steps to manage both effectively. A harmonious balance between restful sleep and stress management is essential for overall mental health and well-being.

The Link Between Sleep and Anxiety Disorders

In our ongoing exploration of the profound connection between sleep and mental health, we now venture into the intricate relationship between sleep and anxiety disorders. Anxiety is a common and challenging mental health condition that can both disrupt sleep and be exacerbated by sleep disturbances.

Sleep and the Anxious Mind

Anxiety and sleep are closely intertwined, and they can either support or undermine each other. Understanding this relationship is crucial for managing anxiety effectively.

Here's how sleep influences anxiety and vice versa:

1. **Sleep Quality and Anxiety:** Poor sleep quality, including difficulty falling asleep, staying asleep, or experiencing restorative sleep, can increase the risk of developing anxiety disorders. Sleep disturbances can heighten emotional reactivity and contribute to feelings of

anxiety.

2. **Anxiety and Sleep Onset:** Anxiety often manifests as racing thoughts, worry, and restlessness, making it challenging to quiet the mind and fall asleep. Individuals with anxiety disorders may experience prolonged sleep onset, leading to sleep deprivation.

3. **Nighttime Anxiety:** Anxiety can disrupt sleep by causing nighttime awakenings and nightmares. This can create a vicious cycle, as sleep disruptions further exacerbate anxiety symptoms.

4. **Emotion Regulation:** Sleep is essential for emotional regulation. Inadequate sleep can lead to increased emotional reactivity, making individuals more susceptible to anxiety symptoms.

5. **Cognitive Function:** Sleep deprivation can impair cognitive function, including concentration and decision-making, which can contribute to feelings of anxiety and stress.

The Impact of Sleep Disruptions on Anxiety Disorders

Chronic sleep disruptions can have significant implications for individuals with anxiety disorders:

1. **Exacerbated Anxiety Symptoms:** Sleep disturbances can worsen anxiety symptoms, leading to increased feelings of worry, fear, and restlessness.

2. **Reduced Treatment Efficacy:** Sleep problems can make it more challenging for individuals with anxiety disorders to respond effectively to treatment, including therapy and medication.

3. **Impaired Quality of Life:** Poor sleep quality can significantly impact an individual's overall quality of life, contributing to a cycle of anxiety and sleep disturbances.

Strategies for Managing Anxiety Through Better Sleep

To manage anxiety through better sleep, consider implementing the following strategies:

1. **Stress Management:** Develop effective stress management

techniques, such as mindfulness meditation, deep breathing exercises, or progressive muscle relaxation, to reduce anxiety levels.

2. **Cognitive Behavioral Therapy (CBT):** CBT for insomnia (CBT-I) is a specialized form of therapy that can help individuals with anxiety-related sleep disturbances. It addresses the thoughts and behaviors that contribute to poor sleep.

3. **Establish a Sleep Routine:** Create a consistent sleep schedule and bedtime routine to signal to your body that it's time to wind down and prepare for rest.

4. **Limit Screen Time:** Avoid screens for at least an hour before bedtime to minimize exposure to stimulating blue light.

5. **Physical Activity:** Engage in regular physical activity, which can help reduce anxiety levels. However, avoid intense workouts close to bedtime, as they can be stimulating.

6. **Nutrition:** Maintain a balanced diet and avoid heavy or spicy meals close to bedtime. Limit caffeine and alcohol intake, especially in the evening.

7. **Sleep Hygiene:** Create a comfortable sleep environment by keeping your bedroom dark, quiet, and at a comfortable temperature.

By recognizing the intricate link between sleep and anxiety disorders, you can take proactive steps to manage anxiety effectively and improve your overall mental health. Quality sleep becomes a valuable tool in breaking the cycle of anxiety and sleep disturbances, fostering a sense of calm and well-being.

Sleep and Depression: Causes and Solutions

In our exploration of the profound connection between sleep and mental health, we now turn our focus to the intricate relationship between sleep and depression. Depression is a complex and challenging mental health condition that often involves disruptions in sleep patterns.

Sleep Disturbances in Depression

Sleep disturbances are a hallmark of depression, and they can manifest in various ways:

1. **Insomnia:** Many individuals with depression experience insomnia, which involves difficulty falling asleep, staying asleep, or waking up too early. This contributes to sleep deprivation and exacerbates depressive symptoms.
2. **Hypersomnia:** Some individuals with depression may experience hypersomnia, characterized by excessive sleepiness and long sleep durations. Despite extended sleep, they often wake up feeling unrefreshed.
3. **Nightmares:** Depression can lead to vivid and distressing nightmares, causing nighttime awakenings and further disrupting sleep.
4. **Sleep Fragmentation:** Individuals with depression often experience fragmented sleep, with frequent awakenings throughout the night. This reduces the quality of sleep and contributes to daytime fatigue.

The Impact of Sleep on Depression

The relationship between sleep and depression is bidirectional. Sleep disturbances can contribute to the development and exacerbation of depression, and depression can worsen sleep problems. Understanding this interplay is essential for managing depression effectively.

Here's how sleep influences depression and vice versa:

1. **Increased Risk:** Chronic sleep disturbances, especially insomnia, increase the risk of developing depression. Sleep problems can precede the onset of depressive symptoms.
2. **Worsened Symptoms:** Poor sleep quality can exacerbate depressive symptoms, leading to increased feelings of sadness, hopelessness, and fatigue.
3. **Reduced Treatment Efficacy:** Sleep problems can make it more challenging for individuals with depression to respond effectively to treatment, including therapy and medication.
4. **Impaired Cognitive Function:** Sleep deprivation impairs cognitive function, including concentration and memory, which can worsen depressive symptoms.

5. **Mood Regulation:** Adequate sleep is crucial for emotional regulation. Sleep-deprived individuals are more susceptible to mood swings and negative emotions.

Strategies for Managing Depression Through Better Sleep

To manage depression through better sleep, consider implementing the following strategies:

1. **Treatment for Depression:** Seek professional help for your depression, including therapy and medication as recommended by a healthcare provider. Treating the underlying depression can often improve sleep.
2. **Cognitive Behavioral Therapy for Insomnia (CBT-I):** CBT-I is a specialized form of therapy that addresses sleep problems. It can be effective for individuals with depression-related sleep disturbances.
3. **Establish a Sleep Routine:** Create a consistent sleep schedule and bedtime routine to signal to your body that it's time to wind down and prepare for rest.
4. **Limit Screen Time:** Avoid screens for at least an hour before bedtime to minimize exposure to stimulating blue light.
5. **Physical Activity:** Engage in regular physical activity, which can help improve sleep quality and mood. However, avoid intense workouts close to bedtime.
6. **Nutrition:** Maintain a balanced diet and avoid heavy or spicy meals close to bedtime. Limit caffeine and alcohol intake, especially in the evening.
7. **Sleep Hygiene:** Create a comfortable sleep environment by keeping your bedroom dark, quiet, and at a comfortable temperature.

By recognizing the complex relationship between sleep and depression, you can take proactive steps to manage depression effectively and improve your overall mental health. Quality sleep becomes a valuable ally in the journey towards recovery and emotional well-being.

Insomnia and Its Effects on Mental Well-being

In our ongoing exploration of the intricate relationship between sleep and mental health, we now delve into the specific sleep disorder of insomnia and its profound effects on mental well-being. Insomnia is a common sleep disorder characterized by persistent difficulty falling asleep, staying asleep, or experiencing restorative sleep. Its impact on mental health is significant, and in this chapter, we'll explore the causes of insomnia, how it affects mental well-being, and strategies for managing insomnia to promote better mental health.

Understanding Insomnia

Insomnia is more than just an occasional night of poor sleep; it's a persistent and distressing sleep disorder that can have far-reaching consequences for mental health. Insomnia can manifest in several ways:

1. **Difficulty Falling Asleep:** Individuals with insomnia may struggle to initiate sleep, often lying awake for extended periods before falling asleep.
2. **Frequent Awakenings:** Those with insomnia may wake up frequently throughout the night, disrupting the continuity of sleep.
3. **Early Morning Awakenings:** Some individuals with insomnia wake up too early in the morning and find it difficult to return to sleep.
4. **Non-Restorative Sleep:** Even if individuals with insomnia spend sufficient time in bed, they often wake up feeling unrefreshed and fatigued.

The Impact of Insomnia on Mental Well-being

Insomnia can have profound effects on mental well-being and is closely linked to several mental health conditions:

1. **Increased Risk of Mood Disorders:** Insomnia is a significant risk factor for mood disorders such as depression and anxiety. Persistent sleep disturbances can exacerbate feelings of sadness and worry.
2. **Cognitive Impairment:** Sleep disruptions caused by insomnia can lead to cognitive impairment, affecting memory, concentration, and

decision-making abilities.

3. **Stress and Anxiety:** Insomnia can increase stress levels and contribute to the development of anxiety disorders. The worry about not being able to sleep can perpetuate the cycle of insomnia.

4. **Reduced Quality of Life:** Chronic insomnia can significantly diminish an individual's quality of life, impacting their ability to function in daily life and enjoy activities.

5. **Daytime Fatigue:** The chronic fatigue resulting from insomnia can lead to decreased energy levels and motivation, further affecting mental well-being.

Strategies for Managing Insomnia and Promoting Mental Health

To manage insomnia and promote better mental health, consider implementing the following strategies:

1. **Cognitive Behavioral Therapy for Insomnia (CBT-I):** CBT-I is a highly effective treatment for insomnia. It addresses the thoughts and behaviors that contribute to sleep problems and helps individuals develop healthier sleep patterns.

2. **Sleep Restriction:** This technique involves limiting time in bed to match actual sleep time, gradually increasing it as sleep improves.

3. **Stimulus Control:** This technique helps individuals associate the bed with sleep rather than wakefulness by establishing a consistent sleep schedule and bedtime routine.

4. **Sleep Hygiene:** Create a comfortable sleep environment by keeping your bedroom dark, quiet, and at a comfortable temperature.

5. **Limit Screen Time:** Avoid screens for at least an hour before bedtime to minimize exposure to stimulating blue light.

6. **Physical Activity:** Engage in regular physical activity, which can improve sleep quality and mental well-being. However, avoid intense workouts close to bedtime.

7. **Nutrition:** Maintain a balanced diet and avoid heavy or spicy meals close to bedtime. Limit caffeine and alcohol intake, especially in the evening.

8. **Stress Management:** Develop effective stress management techniques, such as mindfulness meditation, deep breathing exercises, or progressive muscle relaxation, to reduce anxiety and improve sleep.

By recognizing the profound impact of insomnia on mental well-being and implementing effective strategies for managing it, you can regain control over your sleep and overall mental health. Quality sleep becomes a powerful tool in nurturing emotional well-being and resilience.

Chapter 4: Common Sleep Disorders

Insomnia: Types, Causes, and Treatment Options

As we continue our exploration into the world of sleep and its various facets, we now focus on one of the most prevalent sleep disorders: insomnia. Insomnia is more than just occasional sleepless nights; it's a persistent condition that affects millions of people worldwide.

Understanding Insomnia

Insomnia is a multifaceted sleep disorder characterized by persistent difficulties with falling asleep, staying asleep, or experiencing restorative sleep, despite having the opportunity and desire to sleep. It can manifest in various forms:

1. **Difficulty Falling Asleep:** Onset insomnia involves the inability to initiate sleep when desired, often leading to prolonged periods of wakefulness before finally falling asleep.
2. **Frequent Awakenings:** Middle-of-the-night or maintenance insomnia involves frequent awakenings during the night, disrupting the continuity of sleep.
3. **Early Morning Awakenings:** Terminal insomnia is characterized by waking up too early in the morning and being unable to return to sleep, even when sleep duration has been insufficient.
4. **Non-Restorative Sleep:** Individuals with insomnia may spend adequate time in bed but wake up feeling unrefreshed and fatigued.

Types of Insomnia

Insomnia can be categorized into different types based on its duration:

1. **Transient Insomnia:** Lasting for a few nights or weeks, transient insomnia is often linked to stress, travel, or life changes.
2. **Short-Term Insomnia:** Short-term insomnia persists for several weeks and is typically associated with a specific stressor or event.
3. **Chronic Insomnia:** Chronic insomnia is diagnosed when sleep

disturbances persist for three or more nights a week for at least three months. It may be primary (not linked to other medical or psychological conditions) or secondary (related to other factors).

Causes of Insomnia

Insomnia can have a wide range of causes, including:

1. **Stress and Anxiety:** High levels of stress, anxiety, or worry can make it challenging to relax and fall asleep.
2. **Depression:** Depression is often associated with insomnia, with individuals experiencing difficulty falling asleep, frequent awakenings, or early morning awakenings.
3. **Medical Conditions:** Certain medical conditions, such as chronic pain, respiratory disorders, and gastrointestinal problems, can contribute to insomnia.
4. **Medications:** Some medications, including stimulants, decongestants, and certain antidepressants, can disrupt sleep patterns.
5. **Substance Use:** The use of alcohol, caffeine, or nicotine, particularly close to bedtime, can interfere with sleep.
6. **Poor Sleep Habits:** Irregular sleep schedules, excessive napping, and exposure to screens before bedtime can all contribute to insomnia.

Treatment Options for Insomnia

Fortunately, insomnia is a treatable condition, and various strategies and interventions can help individuals overcome it. Treatment options may include:

1. **Cognitive Behavioral Therapy for Insomnia (CBT-I):** CBT-I is considered the gold standard for treating insomnia. It addresses the thoughts, behaviors, and habits that contribute to sleep problems and helps individuals develop healthier sleep patterns.
2. **Medications:** In some cases, healthcare providers may prescribe sleep medications, such as sedative-hypnotics, for short-term relief of insomnia symptoms. However, these are generally not recommended

for long-term use due to potential side effects and the risk of dependence.

3. **Lifestyle Modifications:** Lifestyle changes, including maintaining a consistent sleep schedule, creating a comfortable sleep environment, and practicing good sleep hygiene, can significantly improve sleep quality.

4. **Stress Management:** Techniques such as mindfulness meditation, progressive muscle relaxation, and deep breathing exercises can help reduce stress and anxiety, making it easier to fall asleep.

5. **Limiting Substance Use:** Reducing or eliminating the consumption of caffeine, nicotine, and alcohol, especially close to bedtime, can improve sleep.

6. **Physical Activity:** Regular physical activity, performed earlier in the day, can promote better sleep quality.

7. **Sleep Education:** Learning about healthy sleep habits and the importance of sleep can empower individuals to take control of their sleep.

By understanding the different types of insomnia, its potential causes, and the various treatment options available, individuals can work toward overcoming this sleep disorder and enjoying restorative, refreshing sleep once again. Insomnia is a common challenge, but with the right strategies and support, it can be effectively managed.

Sleep Apnea: Recognizing Symptoms and Seeking Treatment

Let's dive into another prevalent sleep disorder: sleep apnea. Sleep apnea is a condition characterized by repeated interruptions in breathing during sleep, leading to disrupted sleep patterns and various health concerns. We'll explore the different types of sleep apnea, its symptoms, potential health risks, and the importance of seeking treatment for this potentially serious disorder.

Understanding Sleep Apnea

Sleep apnea is a sleep disorder characterized by periods of interrupted breathing during sleep. The most common types of sleep apnea are:

1. **Obstructive Sleep Apnea (OSA):** This occurs when the muscles in the back of the throat relax excessively, causing a blockage of the airway.
2. **Central Sleep Apnea (CSA):** CSA is less common and is associated with a failure of the brain to transmit the proper signals to the muscles responsible for controlling breathing.
3. **Complex Sleep Apnea Syndrome:** Also known as treatment-emergent central sleep apnea, this is a combination of OSA and CSA.

Recognizing Symptoms of Sleep Apnea

Sleep apnea can have a wide range of symptoms, including:

1. **Loud Snoring:** One of the hallmark signs of sleep apnea, particularly in OSA, is loud and chronic snoring.
2. **Pauses in Breathing:** Witnessed pauses in breathing during sleep, often accompanied by choking or gasping for air.
3. **Excessive Daytime Sleepiness:** Individuals with sleep apnea often experience severe daytime fatigue and excessive sleepiness, even after a full night's sleep.
4. **Morning Headaches:** Frequent morning headaches are a common symptom due to oxygen deprivation during sleep.
5. **Difficulty Concentrating:** Poor sleep quality leads to difficulty concentrating, memory problems, and reduced cognitive function.
6. **Irritability:** Irritability and mood changes can result from chronic sleep disruption.
7. **Frequent Urination at Night:** Nocturia, or the need to urinate frequently during the night, is often associated with sleep apnea.

The Health Risks of Untreated Sleep Apnea

Sleep apnea is not a benign condition; it can have serious health consequences if left untreated:

1. **Cardiovascular Issues:** Sleep apnea is associated with an increased risk of hypertension, heart disease, and stroke due to the strain placed

on the cardiovascular system during apnea episodes.

2. **Type 2 Diabetes:** The disrupted sleep patterns and altered metabolism associated with sleep apnea can contribute to the development of type 2 diabetes.

3. **Daytime Accidents:** Severe daytime sleepiness can lead to an increased risk of accidents, including motor vehicle accidents.

4. **Mood Disorders:** Sleep apnea can exacerbate or contribute to mood disorders such as depression and anxiety.

5. **Reduced Quality of Life:** Poor sleep quality can significantly impact an individual's quality of life, affecting their physical and emotional well-being.

Seeking Treatment for Sleep Apnea

Recognizing the symptoms of sleep apnea and seeking treatment is crucial for improving sleep quality and reducing health risks. Treatment options for sleep apnea may include:

1. **Continuous Positive Airway Pressure (CPAP):** This is the most common and effective treatment for OSA. It involves wearing a mask over the nose or nose and mouth, delivering pressurized air to keep the airway open during sleep.

2. **Bi-level Positive Airway Pressure (BiPAP):** Similar to CPAP, BiPAP delivers two levels of air pressure: a higher pressure during inhalation and a lower pressure during exhalation.

3. **Oral Appliances:** These devices are designed to reposition the jaw and tongue to keep the airway open during sleep, suitable for mild to moderate OSA.

4. **Lifestyle Changes:** Weight loss, avoiding alcohol and sedatives, and sleeping on your side can help reduce the severity of sleep apnea symptoms.

5. **Surgery:** In some cases, surgical procedures may be recommended to address physical obstructions in the airway.

By recognizing the symptoms of sleep apnea and seeking appropriate treatment, individuals can significantly improve their sleep quality, reduce health risks, and enhance their overall well-being. Sleep apnea is a treatable condition, and with the right interventions, individuals can enjoy more restful and uninterrupted sleep.

Narcolepsy: Understanding Sudden Sleep Attacks

We'll explore narcolepsy, a unique and often misunderstood sleep disorder. Narcolepsy is characterized by excessive daytime sleepiness and sudden, uncontrollable sleep attacks. We'll delve into the symptoms, underlying causes, impact on daily life, and potential treatment options for individuals living with narcolepsy.

The Enigma of Narcolepsy

Narcolepsy is a neurological sleep disorder that disrupts the normal sleep-wake cycle. It is often misunderstood and can have a significant impact on an individual's life.

Symptoms of Narcolepsy

Narcolepsy is marked by several hallmark symptoms:

1. **Excessive Daytime Sleepiness:** People with narcolepsy experience extreme daytime fatigue, which can make it difficult to stay awake and alert.
2. **Cataplexy:** Cataplexy is the sudden loss of muscle control, often triggered by strong emotions like laughter or anger. It can range from mild muscle weakness to complete collapse.
3. **Sleep Attacks:** Narcoleptic sleep attacks are episodes of sudden and irresistible sleepiness. These can occur at any time, regardless of the individual's level of alertness or activity.
4. **Sleep Paralysis:** Individuals with narcolepsy may experience sleep paralysis, a temporary inability to move or speak while falling asleep or waking up.
5. **Hallucinations:** Vivid and often frightening dream-like experiences,

known as hypnagogic hallucinations when falling asleep or hypnopompic hallucinations when waking up, are common in narcolepsy.

Understanding the Causes

Narcolepsy is primarily a neurological disorder, with most cases attributed to a deficiency of hypocretin, a neurotransmitter that regulates wakefulness and sleep. The exact cause of hypocretin deficiency is still under investigation, but it is believed to involve an autoimmune response.

Daily Life with Narcolepsy

Living with narcolepsy presents unique challenges:

1. **Work and Education:** Maintaining a consistent work or school schedule can be challenging due to sudden sleep attacks and excessive daytime sleepiness.
2. **Social Interactions:** Coping with cataplexy and managing sleepiness in social situations can be emotionally taxing.
3. **Driving and Safety:** People with narcolepsy must take precautions when driving or operating machinery due to the risk of sleep attacks.
4. **Mood and Mental Health:** Narcolepsy can lead to feelings of frustration, isolation, and depression, particularly when symptoms are severe.

Treatment Options

While narcolepsy cannot be cured, treatment options are available to manage its symptoms:

1. **Stimulant Medications:** Stimulants like modafinil or methylphenidate can help improve wakefulness and alertness during the day.
2. **Antidepressant Medications:** Certain antidepressants, such as selective serotonin and norepinephrine reuptake inhibitors (SSRIs and SNRIs), may help manage cataplexy and other symptoms.

3. **Sodium Oxybate:** This medication can improve sleep quality at night and reduce daytime sleepiness.
4. **Lifestyle Adjustments:** Establishing regular sleep patterns, taking short planned naps, and avoiding alcohol and caffeine close to bedtime can help manage symptoms.
5. **Support and Education:** Joining support groups and educating oneself and loved ones about narcolepsy can provide valuable emotional and practical support.

Conclusion

Narcolepsy is a complex sleep disorder that affects every aspect of a person's life. Understanding its symptoms, causes, and potential treatments is essential for those living with narcolepsy and for promoting awareness and empathy in society at large. With appropriate treatment and support, individuals with narcolepsy can lead fulfilling lives despite the unique challenges posed by this condition.

Restless Legs Syndrome (RLS) and Periodic Limb Movement Disorder (PLMD)

These conditions can lead to restless nights, chronic sleep disturbances, and daytime fatigue. We'll explore the symptoms, causes, and potential treatments for both RLS and PLMD.

Restless Legs Syndrome (RLS)

Understanding RLS

Restless Legs Syndrome, often abbreviated as RLS, is a neurological disorder characterized by an irresistible urge to move the legs, typically during periods of rest or inactivity, especially in the evening and at night. This condition can disrupt sleep and negatively impact a person's quality of life.

Symptoms of RLS

RLS is often associated with the following symptoms:

1. **Unpleasant Sensations:** People with RLS describe uncomfortable sensations in their legs, often described as crawling, tingling, burning, or itching.
2. **Urge to Move:** The sensations in the legs are accompanied by a strong urge to move them, which provides temporary relief from the discomfort.
3. **Worsening in the Evening:** RLS symptoms tend to worsen in the evening and at night, making it difficult to relax and fall asleep.

Causes and Triggers

The exact cause of RLS is not fully understood, but several factors may contribute, including:

1. **Genetics:** RLS can run in families, suggesting a genetic component.
2. **Iron Deficiency:** Low iron levels in the brain may play a role in RLS, making iron supplementation a potential treatment option.
3. **Pregnancy:** Some women experience RLS during pregnancy, especially in the third trimester.

Treatment for RLS

Treatment options for RLS may include:

1. **Lifestyle Changes:** Managing caffeine and alcohol intake, regular exercise, and practicing good sleep hygiene can help alleviate symptoms.
2. **Medications:** Medications such as dopamine agonists, alpha-2 delta calcium channel ligands, and opioids may be prescribed to relieve symptoms.

Periodic Limb Movement Disorder (PLMD)

Understanding PLMD

Periodic Limb Movement Disorder, or PLMD, is a sleep disorder characterized by repetitive, involuntary, and stereotypical limb movements, typically involving the legs. These movements occur during sleep and can disrupt the sleep cycle, leading to poor sleep quality.

Symptoms of PLMD

The primary symptom of PLMD is the repetitive and periodic movement of the legs during sleep, often involving flexing and extending of the toes, ankles, knees, or hips. These movements can occur throughout the night, occurring at regular intervals, and are often accompanied by brief awakenings.

Causes and Triggers

PLMD can have various causes and may be associated with other medical conditions, including:

1. **Iron Deficiency:** Like RLS, PLMD may be linked to low iron levels in the brain.
2. **Neurological Conditions:** PLMD can occur in conjunction with neurological conditions such as Parkinson's disease or neuropathy.

Treatment for PLMD

Treatment options for PLMD may include:

1. **Medications:** Medications that increase dopamine levels in the brain, such as dopamine agonists, may help reduce limb movements and improve sleep quality.
2. **Iron Supplementation:** If iron deficiency is identified, iron supplements may be recommended.

Parasomnias: Sleepwalking, Night Terrors, and REM Sleep Behavior Disorder

These disorders involve unusual and often disruptive behaviors or experiences during sleep. We will explore three common parasomnias: sleepwalking, night terrors, and REM Sleep Behavior Disorder (RBD), discussing their symptoms, potential causes, and management strategies.

Understanding Parasomnias

Parasomnias are a category of sleep disorders characterized by abnormal behaviors, movements, emotions, perceptions, or dreams during sleep. They can occur during any stage of sleep and often disrupt both the individual experiencing the parasomnia and their sleep partners.

Sleepwalking (Somnambulism)

Symptoms of Sleepwalking

Sleepwalking, or somnambulism, involves a person getting out of bed and engaging in various activities while still asleep. These activities can range from simple tasks like walking around the room to more complex behaviors like cooking or even driving. Sleepwalkers often have no memory of their actions.

Causes of Sleepwalking

The exact cause of sleepwalking is not fully understood, but it may be influenced by various factors, including genetics, sleep deprivation, stress, and certain medications. Sleepwalking is more common in children but can persist into adulthood.

Management of Sleepwalking

Managing sleepwalking typically involves creating a safe sleep environment to prevent injury. Locking doors and windows, removing obstacles, and installing gates or alarms can help. In some cases, addressing underlying factors like stress or sleep deprivation may reduce the frequency of sleepwalking episodes.

Night Terrors (Sleep Terrors)

Symptoms of Night Terrors

Night terrors, or sleep terrors, are intense episodes of fear, screaming, and intense agitation during sleep. These episodes typically occur during non-REM (NREM) sleep, often in the first half of the night. Unlike nightmares, individuals experiencing night terrors are usually not aware of their surroundings and cannot recall the event upon waking.

Causes of Night Terrors

Night terrors are most common in children and tend to decrease with age. They can be triggered by factors such as fever, sleep deprivation, stress, and certain medications.

Management of Night Terrors

Night terrors often do not require treatment, especially in children, as they tend to outgrow them. However, if night terrors are frequent or cause significant distress, a healthcare provider may explore treatment options, which may include addressing underlying factors, such as sleep deprivation.

REM Sleep Behavior Disorder (RBD)

Symptoms of RBD

RBD is a parasomnia characterized by the acting out of vivid and often violent dreams during REM (rapid eye movement) sleep. Individuals with RBD may talk, shout, kick, punch, or even physically enact the content of their dreams, potentially injuring themselves or their sleep partners.

Causes of RBD

RBD is often associated with neurodegenerative conditions like Parkinson's disease and may be an early sign of such conditions. It can also occur independently without an underlying neurological disorder.

Management of RBD

Treatment for RBD typically involves addressing the underlying cause, if present. In cases where RBD is not associated with a neurological condition, medication may be prescribed to suppress dream-enacting behaviors and prevent injuries during sleep.

Chapter 5: Sleep Hygiene and Environment

Creating the Ideal Sleep Environment: Dark, Quiet, and Comfortable

Creating the perfect sleep environment is key to achieving restful and restorative sleep. We'll explore how to make your bedroom a sanctuary for sleep by optimizing its darkness, tranquility, and comfort.

The Importance of a Sleep-Conducive Environment

Creating the right sleep environment can significantly impact your sleep quality and overall well-being. An optimal sleep environment promotes relaxation, reduces disturbances, and sets the stage for restorative rest.

1. Darkness: The Key to Melatonin Production

Why Darkness Matters

Darkness is essential for the production of melatonin, a hormone that regulates your sleep-wake cycle. Exposure to light, especially blue light emitted by screens, suppresses melatonin production, making it harder to fall asleep and stay asleep.

How to Achieve Darkness

1. **Use Blackout Curtains:** Install blackout curtains or shades to block out external light sources, such as streetlights or the morning sun.
2. **Cover Electronic Displays:** Cover or turn off electronic displays like clocks or devices that emit light.
3. **Limit Screen Time:** Avoid screens (phones, tablets, computers, TVs) for at least an hour before bedtime, and consider using blue light filters on electronic devices.
4. **Invest in an Eye Mask:** If you can't eliminate all sources of light, a comfortable eye mask can provide complete darkness.

2. Quiet: A Peaceful Sleep Oasis

Why Quietness Matters

A quiet sleep environment is crucial for minimizing disturbances that can disrupt your sleep cycles. Sudden noises or constant background noise can interfere with your ability to fall asleep and stay asleep.

How to Create Quietness

1. **Earplugs:** Invest in high-quality earplugs to reduce noise disruptions from the surrounding environment.
2. **White Noise Machines:** Consider using white noise machines or apps that produce consistent background noise, which can help drown out intermittent sounds.
3. **Soundproofing:** If possible, add soundproofing materials to your bedroom walls or windows to reduce external noise.
4. **Communicate:** If you share your sleeping space, communicate with your bed partner about noise-related concerns and find solutions together.

3. Comfort: The Right Bed and Bedding

Why Comfort Matters

A comfortable sleep environment ensures that you can relax physically and mentally. Your bed and bedding play a significant role in promoting comfort.

How to Achieve Comfort

1. **Quality Mattress and Pillows:** Invest in a comfortable mattress and pillows that provide the right level of support for your body.
2. **Bedding Materials:** Choose bedding materials (sheets, blankets, and comforters) that feel comfortable against your skin and maintain a comfortable temperature.
3. **Temperature Control:** Maintain a comfortable room temperature by using fans or adjusting the thermostat to your preferred setting.
4. **Declutter:** Keep your sleep space free of clutter and distractions to promote relaxation.

By optimizing the darkness, tranquility, and comfort of your sleep environment, you can create a sanctuary for restorative sleep. Remember that everyone's preferences may vary, so it's essential to customize your sleep environment to suit your individual needs and preferences. A peaceful sleep environment sets the stage for a night of rejuvenating rest and contributes to your overall well-being.

The Importance of a Consistent Sleep Schedule

Establishing and adhering to a regular sleep schedule can significantly impact your sleep quality, overall health, and daily functioning. We'll explore why consistency matters and how to cultivate a steady sleep routine.

The Significance of a Consistent Sleep Schedule

Consistency in your sleep schedule involves going to bed and waking up at the same times every day, even on weekends. This routine aligns your body's internal clock, known as the circadian rhythm, with your desired sleep pattern. Here's why it's crucial:

1. Regulates Your Circadian Rhythm

Your circadian rhythm is a natural, internal clock that regulates various biological processes, including sleep-wake cycles. Consistent sleep schedules help synchronize your circadian rhythm, making it easier to fall asleep and wake up at the desired times.

2. Enhances Sleep Quality

A regular sleep schedule promotes more restful and uninterrupted sleep. When your body knows when to expect sleep, it can enter deep, restorative sleep stages more efficiently.

3. Improves Sleep Efficiency

Consistency helps improve sleep efficiency, which is the ratio of time spent asleep to the total time spent in bed. With a steady schedule, you're less likely to spend extended periods awake in bed, reducing the risk of insomnia.

4. Enhances Alertness and Cognitive Function

A consistent sleep routine ensures you wake up feeling refreshed and alert. This can lead to improved cognitive function, better concentration, and increased daytime productivity.

5. Supports Physical and Mental Health

Regular sleep patterns are associated with better physical and mental health outcomes. Disruptions to your sleep schedule can contribute to mood disorders, such as depression and anxiety, and increase the risk of chronic conditions like obesity and diabetes.

How to Establish and Maintain a Consistent Sleep Schedule

Creating a consistent sleep schedule involves more than just setting a bedtime and wake-up time. Here's a step-by-step guide:

1. **Determine Your Ideal Sleep Duration:** Calculate the amount of sleep you need each night, typically between 7 to 9 hours for adults.
2. **Set Fixed Bedtimes and Wake-Up Times:** Choose specific times to go to bed and wake up, and stick to them every day, even on weekends.
3. **Gradual Adjustments:** If your current schedule differs significantly from your desired one, make gradual adjustments, moving bedtime and wake-up time by 15-30 minutes each night until you reach your goal.
4. **Create a Wind-Down Routine:** Develop a relaxing bedtime routine that signals to your body that it's time to sleep. Activities like reading, taking a warm bath, or practicing relaxation techniques can be part of your wind-down routine.
5. **Limit Exposure to Screens:** Avoid screens (phones, tablets, computers, TVs) at least an hour before bedtime to minimize exposure to stimulating blue light.
6. **Control Light Exposure:** Ensure your sleep environment is dark when it's time to sleep and exposed to natural light during the day to reinforce your circadian rhythm.

7. **Stay Consistent on Weekends:** Try to maintain your sleep schedule even on weekends to avoid "social jetlag," which can disrupt your rhythm.

8. **Monitor and Adjust:** Regularly assess your sleep quality and make adjustments if necessary. If you're consistently getting enough sleep but still feel tired during the day, consult a healthcare provider for further evaluation.

By prioritizing a consistent sleep schedule, you can optimize your sleep patterns, enhance your overall health and well-being, and enjoy the benefits of restorative sleep on a daily basis.

The Role of Diet and Nutrition in Sleep Quality

What you eat and drink can significantly impact your sleep patterns and overall well-being. We'll delve into the foods and beverages that can either promote or hinder restful sleep and provide tips on how to make dietary choices that contribute to better sleep quality.

The Link Between Diet and Sleep

The relationship between diet and sleep is intricate and bidirectional. Your dietary choices can influence your sleep quality, and your sleep patterns can, in turn, affect your food preferences and eating habits. Here's why paying attention to your diet is essential for better sleep:

1. Timing Matters:

- **Meal Timing:** Eating large, heavy meals close to bedtime can lead to discomfort and indigestion, making it harder to fall asleep. Aim to finish your last substantial meal at least two to three hours before bedtime.
- **Snacking:** While it's generally advisable to avoid heavy meals before sleep, light, balanced snacks containing sleep-promoting nutrients like complex carbohydrates and tryptophan can be beneficial.

2. The Impact of Food Choices:

- **Sleep-Promoting Nutrients:** Certain nutrients can enhance sleep quality. These include:

- **Tryptophan:** Found in foods like turkey, chicken, nuts, and seeds, tryptophan is a precursor to the sleep-inducing hormone melatonin.
- **Magnesium:** Magnesium-rich foods like leafy greens, nuts, and whole grains can help relax muscles and improve sleep quality.
- **Complex Carbohydrates:** Foods like whole grains, sweet potatoes, and legumes can help regulate blood sugar levels and promote steady sleep.

- **Caffeine and Alcohol:** Both caffeine and alcohol can disrupt sleep. Caffeine is a stimulant that should be avoided several hours before bedtime, and while alcohol may initially make you feel drowsy, it can disrupt the sleep cycle, leading to fragmented sleep.
- **Spicy and Acidic Foods:** Spicy and acidic foods can cause heartburn and indigestion, which can interfere with sleep.

3. Hydration and Sleep:

- **Fluid Intake:** While it's important to stay hydrated, excessive fluid intake in the hours leading up to bedtime may lead to frequent awakenings during the night to use the bathroom. Aim to hydrate earlier in the day and reduce fluid intake closer to bedtime.

4. The Role of Sugar:

- **Sugar and Sleep:** High-sugar diets are associated with poor sleep quality. Excess sugar intake can lead to fluctuations in blood sugar levels and disrupt sleep patterns.

5. Individual Variation:

- **Personal Sensitivity:** It's important to recognize that individual responses to specific foods and beverages can vary. Pay attention to how different foods and drinks affect your sleep and make adjustments accordingly.

Tips for Promoting Better Sleep Through Diet:

1. **Balanced Dinner:** Opt for a balanced dinner that includes lean proteins, complex carbohydrates, and vegetables. Avoid large, heavy meals close to bedtime.
2. **Snack Wisely:** If you need a bedtime snack, choose foods that contain tryptophan, such as a small turkey sandwich or a banana with nut butter.
3. **Limit Caffeine and Alcohol:** Reduce caffeine intake in the afternoon and evening, and be mindful of alcohol consumption, especially close to bedtime.
4. **Stay Hydrated:** Stay adequately hydrated throughout the day, but cut back on fluid intake in the hours before bedtime.
5. **Mindful Eating:** Pay attention to how specific foods affect your sleep, and make dietary choices that support your sleep goals.

By recognizing the profound influence of diet and nutrition on sleep quality, you can make informed choices that contribute to better sleep patterns and overall well-being. Implementing healthy eating habits and timing your meals wisely can positively impact the duration and quality of your sleep, enhancing your daily life and productivity.

The Impact of Technology on Sleep: Tips for a Digital Detox

The ever-present screens of smartphones, tablets, computers, and televisions have become integral to modern life but can also disrupt our sleep patterns. We'll discuss the impact of technology on sleep and share strategies to create a healthier balance between our digital lives and restful sleep.

The Technology-Sleep Connection

The proliferation of digital devices and the constant connectivity to the internet have changed the way we live and work, but they have also introduced new challenges to our sleep patterns. Here's how technology can impact your sleep:

1. Blue Light Exposure:

- **Blue Light Emission:** Digital screens emit blue light, which can interfere with your body's natural production of melatonin, the hormone that regulates sleep-wake cycles. Exposure to blue light in the evening can make it harder to fall asleep.

2. Sleep Disruption:

- **Stimulation and Distraction:** Scrolling through social media, watching videos, or playing games on screens can be mentally stimulating and lead to bedtime procrastination, delaying the onset of sleep.
- **Notification Disturbances:** The pings, dings, and vibrations of notifications can disrupt sleep by causing awakenings during the night.

3. Mental and Emotional Effects:

- **Stress and Anxiety:** Constant connectivity can contribute to stress and anxiety, which may manifest as racing thoughts when trying to sleep.
- **Comparison and FOMO:** Social media can foster feelings of inadequacy or the fear of missing out (FOMO), which can affect sleep by creating emotional turmoil.

Tips for a Digital Detox to Improve Sleep:

1. **Establish Digital Curfews:**
   - Set a specific time each evening to turn off or put away digital devices. Ideally, this should be at least an hour before bedtime.
2. **Use Night Mode and Blue Light Filters:**
   - Enable night mode or blue light filters on your devices to reduce blue light exposure in the evening.
3. **Create a Charging Station Outside the Bedroom:**
   - Keep your bedroom a screen-free zone by charging devices outside the sleeping area.

4. **Disable Non-Essential Notifications:**
   - Turn off non-essential notifications or set your devices to "Do Not Disturb" mode during your designated sleep hours.
5. **Establish a Bedtime Routine:**
   - Develop a relaxing bedtime routine that doesn't involve screens. Activities like reading, gentle stretching, or meditation can help signal to your body that it's time to wind down.
6. **Limit Screen Time During the Day:**
   - Reduce excessive screen time during the day to minimize overstimulation.
7. **Designate Tech-Free Zones:**
   - Create specific areas in your home, such as the dining room or living room, where screens are not allowed.
8. **Practice Mindfulness:**
   - Be mindful of your digital habits and how they affect your sleep. Identify situations that lead to excessive screen time and work on finding healthier alternatives.
9. **Replace Digital Alarm Clocks:**
   - Use a traditional alarm clock instead of your smartphone as your alarm to avoid the temptation of checking notifications.
10. **Seek Professional Help If Needed:**
    - If technology addiction or the impact of digital devices on your sleep is a persistent problem, consider seeking professional guidance or therapy.

By implementing these strategies and embracing a digital detox, you can strike a healthier balance between technology and sleep. Reducing digital distractions and screen time in the hours leading up to bedtime can lead to improved sleep quality, better overall well-being, and a more peaceful and restorative night's sleep.

Relaxation Techniques and Mindfulness for Better Sleep

In our fast-paced and often stressful lives, the ability to unwind and calm the mind is essential for achieving restful sleep. We'll delve into various relaxation methods and mindfulness exercises that can help you prepare your body and mind for a peaceful night's rest.

The Importance of Relaxation and Mindfulness for Sleep

Stress, anxiety, and racing thoughts can all disrupt your ability to fall asleep and stay asleep. Incorporating relaxation and mindfulness practices into your bedtime routine can help quiet the mind, reduce stress, and promote restorative sleep. Here's why it matters:

1. Stress Reduction:

- **Cortisol Levels:** Chronic stress can lead to elevated cortisol levels, which interfere with sleep. Relaxation and mindfulness can lower stress hormones.

2. Anxiety Management:

- **Anxiety and Sleep:** Persistent anxiety can cause sleep disturbances. Mindfulness practices help manage anxious thoughts and promote relaxation.

3. Improved Sleep Quality:

- **Transition to Sleep:** Relaxation techniques can facilitate the transition from wakefulness to sleep, leading to more restful nights.

4. Sleep-Onset Insomnia:

- **Difficulty Falling Asleep:** If you struggle to fall asleep quickly, relaxation exercises can speed up the process.

5. Sleep Maintenance Insomnia:

- **Waking Up During the Night:** For those who wake up frequently during the night, relaxation and mindfulness can help you return to sleep more easily.

Relaxation Techniques for Better Sleep:

1. **Progressive Muscle Relaxation:** This involves systematically tensing and then relaxing different muscle groups to release physical tension and promote relaxation.
2. **Deep Breathing Exercises:** Deep, slow breaths can calm the nervous system and reduce stress. Try inhaling for a count of four, holding for four, and exhaling for eight.
3. **Guided Imagery:** Visualization exercises take your mind to a peaceful and calming place, diverting attention away from stressors.
4. **Autogenic Training:** This technique involves repeating a series of self-statements focused on promoting relaxation and reducing stress.

Mindfulness Practices for Better Sleep:

1. **Mindful Breathing:** Pay attention to your breath, focusing on each inhale and exhale. When your mind wanders, gently bring it back to your breath.
2. **Body Scan:** Mentally scan your body from head to toe, noticing any areas of tension or discomfort and allowing them to release.
3. **Mindful Meditation:** Dedicate time to sitting in stillness and observing your thoughts without judgment. This practice can help quiet a racing mind.
4. **Yoga Nidra:** Also known as "yogic sleep," this practice involves a guided meditation that induces a state of deep relaxation and promotes restful sleep.

Incorporating Relaxation and Mindfulness into Your Bedtime Routine:

1. **Schedule Relaxation Time:** Set aside time before bed to practice relaxation or mindfulness. Even just 10-15 minutes can be effective.
2. **Create a Calming Environment:** Dim the lights, use soothing colors, and play calming music or nature sounds if they help you relax.
3. **Limit Stimulants:** Avoid caffeine, alcohol, and heavy meals close to bedtime.
4. **Unplug from Screens:** Turn off electronic devices at least an hour

before bedtime to reduce mental stimulation.

5. **Develop a Routine:** Consistency is key. Incorporate relaxation and mindfulness practices into your nightly routine to signal to your body that it's time to wind down.

By embracing relaxation techniques and mindfulness practices, you can reduce the impact of stress and anxiety on your sleep, quiet your mind, and set the stage for a peaceful and rejuvenating night's rest. These practices can become valuable tools in your journey towards better sleep and overall well-being.

Chapter 6: Sleep Across the Lifespan

Sleep in Infants and Children: Developmental Changes and Challenges

Sleep patterns and challenges evolve significantly as children grow and develop. We'll delve into the unique sleep needs of each age group, common sleep issues faced by parents, and strategies to promote healthy sleep in children.

Sleep in Infants (0-12 Months)

Developmental Milestones:

- **Newborns (0-3 Months):** Newborns sleep in short cycles, waking every 2-4 hours to eat. They have no fixed sleep schedule.
- **Infants (3-12 Months):** As infants grow, they gradually establish more regular sleep patterns. Naps become more structured, and nighttime sleep duration typically extends.

Challenges:

- **Frequent Night Wakings:** Newborns need to eat frequently, leading to interrupted sleep for parents.
- **Sleep Regression:** Around 4 months, some infants experience sleep regression, where they may wake more frequently and have trouble self-soothing.

Strategies:

- **Establish a Bedtime Routine:** Create a calming bedtime routine to signal it's time for sleep.
- **Safe Sleep Practices:** Follow safe sleep guidelines, including placing infants on their backs in a crib with no loose bedding.
- **Consistent Sleep Environment:** Keep the sleep environment consistent and comfortable.

Sleep in Toddlers and Preschoolers (1-5 Years)

Developmental Milestones:

- **Toddlers (1-2 Years):** Transition from two naps to one nap. Sleep duration typically ranges from 11-14 hours.
- **Preschoolers (3-5 Years):** One nap is common, with nighttime sleep duration averaging 10-13 hours.

Challenges:

- **Resistance to Bedtime:** Toddlers may resist bedtime, leading to bedtime battles.
- **Nightmares and Night Terrors:** Vivid dreams, nightmares, and night terrors may begin during this age.

Strategies:

- **Consistent Bedtime Routine:** Maintain a consistent bedtime routine to establish healthy sleep habits.
- **Limit Screen Time:** Reduce exposure to screens before bedtime.
- **Address Fears:** Offer comfort and reassurance if children experience nightmares or night terrors.

Sleep in School-Age Children (6-12 Years)

Developmental Milestones:

- **School-Age (6-12 Years):** Most school-age children need 9-12 hours of sleep per night.

Challenges:

- **Overcommitment:** Overscheduling and extracurricular activities can lead to sleep deprivation.
- **Screen Time:** Increased access to screens can disrupt sleep if not

managed.

Strategies:

- **Consistent Bedtime:** Maintain a consistent bedtime routine, even as schedules become busier.
- **Limit Screens Before Bed:** Establish a screen curfew to allow for wind-down time before sleep.

Sleep in Adolescents (13-18 Years)

Developmental Milestones:

- **Adolescents (13-18 Years):** The biological shift in circadian rhythms can lead to delayed sleep patterns. Teens typically require 8-10 hours of sleep.

Challenges:

- **Early School Start Times:** Many schools start early, making it difficult for adolescents to get enough sleep.
- **Peer Pressure and Social Activities:** Social activities and extracurricular commitments can lead to late nights.

Strategies:

- **Advocate for Healthy School Start Times:** Advocate for later school start times to align with adolescent sleep needs.
- **Establish a Consistent Sleep Schedule:** Encourage a consistent sleep schedule, even on weekends.

Understanding the changing sleep needs and challenges faced by children at different stages of development is crucial for parents and caregivers. By implementing appropriate sleep strategies and fostering healthy sleep habits from infancy through adolescence, parents can support their children's physical and cognitive development and set the stage for a lifetime of good sleep hygiene.

Teenagers and Sleep: Balancing School, Social Life, and Rest

Adolescence is a period of significant change, both biologically and socially, and understanding how to promote healthy sleep habits in teenagers is essential for their well-being.

Teenage Sleep Patterns and Challenges

During adolescence, significant changes occur in a teenager's sleep patterns due to shifts in their biological clock, increased academic demands, and active social lives. Here are some key considerations:

1. Biological Shifts:

- **Delayed Sleep Phase:** Adolescents experience a shift in their circadian rhythms, often leading to a preference for later bedtimes and wake times. This is a natural part of adolescent development.

2. Academic Demands:

- **Early School Start Times:** Many schools start early, making it challenging for teenagers to get enough sleep. This misalignment between school schedules and circadian rhythms can result in sleep deprivation.
- **Homework and Study Pressure:** Increasing academic demands, including homework and exam preparation, can encroach on sleep time.

3. Social Activities:

- **Peer and Social Pressure:** Teenagers often engage in social activities, which can extend into late hours, further compromising sleep.

4. Technology: The use of screens, including smartphones and computers, can lead to late-night texting, social media browsing, or gaming, affecting sleep quality.

Balancing Sleep with School and Social Life

Promoting healthy sleep habits in teenagers involves addressing these challenges while recognizing the importance of adequate rest. Here are some strategies for achieving that balance:

1. Advocate for Later School Start Times:

- Encourage schools to consider later start times to better align with teenagers' natural circadian rhythms.

2. Establish a Consistent Sleep Schedule:

- Encourage teenagers to maintain a consistent sleep schedule, even on weekends, to regulate their internal clocks.

3. Limit Screen Time Before Bed:

- Create a "screen curfew" by turning off electronic devices at least an hour before bedtime to minimize the impact of blue light on sleep.

4. Time Management and Prioritization:

- Teach teenagers time management skills to balance academic responsibilities and allocate time for adequate sleep.

5. Create a Relaxing Bedtime Routine:

- Encourage relaxation techniques before bed, such as reading, deep breathing, or meditation, to signal to the body that it's time to wind down.

6. Foster Open Communication:

- Maintain open communication with teenagers about the importance of sleep and the potential consequences of sleep deprivation.

7. Model Healthy Sleep Habits:

- Set an example by prioritizing your own sleep and creating a sleep-conducive environment at home.

8. Encourage Naps:

- If possible, allow for short naps during the day to compensate for lost nighttime sleep.

Balancing the demands of school, social life, and rest can be challenging for teenagers, but it's essential for their overall well-being. By advocating for sleep-friendly school policies, teaching time management skills, and fostering good sleep habits, parents, educators, and caregivers can help teenagers navigate this critical stage of development with the energy and focus they need to succeed.

Sleep During Pregnancy: Coping with Changes in Sleep Patterns

Pregnancy brings about a multitude of physical and hormonal changes that can significantly affect a woman's sleep patterns. We'll discuss these changes, common sleep disturbances during pregnancy, and practical strategies to cope with them for a more restful and comfortable experience.

Sleep Changes During Pregnancy

Pregnancy is a time of profound physiological and hormonal changes, and these changes can have a notable impact on sleep patterns. Understanding these shifts is crucial for expectant mothers:

1. First Trimester (Weeks 1-12):

- **Fatigue:** Many women experience increased fatigue during the first trimester, often needing more daytime naps.
- **Frequent Urination:** Hormonal changes lead to increased blood flow to the kidneys, resulting in more frequent urination, particularly at night.
- **Morning Sickness:** Nausea and vomiting can disrupt sleep, especially in the early hours.

2. Second Trimester (Weeks 13-27):

- **Increased Energy:** Some women experience a temporary boost in energy during this period, leading to more consistent sleep.
- **Growing Discomfort:** As the baby grows, physical discomfort may increase, particularly in the form of back pain and heartburn, which can disrupt sleep.

3. Third Trimester (Weeks 28-40):

- **Frequent Waking:** The need to urinate and increased discomfort can lead to frequent awakenings during the night.
- **Restless Legs Syndrome (RLS):** Some pregnant women experience RLS symptoms, which can interfere with falling asleep.
- **Breathing Challenges:** As the baby grows, there may be increased pressure on the diaphragm, making it more challenging to breathe comfortably when lying down.

Coping with Sleep Changes During Pregnancy

While it's common to experience sleep disturbances during pregnancy, there are strategies to help manage these challenges and improve sleep quality:

1. Establish a Comfortable Sleep Environment:

- Use pillows to support your growing belly and find a comfortable sleeping position, such as sleeping on your left side to improve blood flow to the baby and reduce pressure on major blood vessels.

2. Manage Heartburn:

- Avoid heavy, spicy, or acidic meals close to bedtime to minimize the risk of heartburn. Consider sleeping with your upper body slightly elevated.

3. Stay Hydrated During the Day:

- Drink plenty of fluids early in the day and reduce intake in the evening to minimize nighttime trips to the bathroom.

4. Practice Relaxation Techniques:

- Engage in relaxation exercises such as deep breathing or prenatal yoga to reduce stress and anxiety.

5. Nap When Needed:

- Take short naps during the day to combat fatigue but avoid excessive daytime sleep that might interfere with nighttime sleep.

6. Communicate with Your Healthcare Provider:

- Discuss sleep disturbances with your healthcare provider to rule out any underlying medical concerns.

7. Prepare for Labor and Motherhood:

- Use this time to develop good sleep habits that can be beneficial when caring for a newborn.

Sleep in Older Adults: Understanding Age-Related Sleep Issues

Aging brings about changes in sleep patterns and sleep needs, and it's essential to understand these changes to promote healthy sleep and overall well-being in the elderly. We'll discuss the impact of aging on sleep, common sleep issues in older adults, and strategies to address them.

Aging and Sleep

Aging is associated with several changes in sleep patterns and sleep architecture:

1. Changes in Sleep Architecture:

- **Reduced Deep Sleep:** Older adults often experience a decrease in deep, restorative sleep stages, such as slow-wave sleep (SWS).
- **More Frequent Awakenings:** Aging can lead to more frequent awakenings during the night, reducing overall sleep efficiency.

2. Shifts in Circadian Rhythms:

- **Advanced Sleep Phase:** Older adults may experience an advanced sleep phase, leading to earlier bedtimes and wake times.
- **Phase Delay:** Some older adults may experience a phase delay, making it harder to fall asleep and wake up at the desired times.

3. Sleep Disorders:

- **Insomnia:** Insomnia becomes more common with age, characterized by difficulty falling asleep, staying asleep, or waking up too early.
- **Sleep Apnea:** The risk of sleep apnea increases with age, leading to interrupted breathing during sleep.
- **Restless Legs Syndrome (RLS):** RLS symptoms may worsen in older age, leading to discomfort and sleep disruptions.

4. Medications and Health Conditions:

- Medications and underlying health conditions can contribute to sleep disturbances in older adults.

Coping with Age-Related Sleep Issues

Promoting healthy sleep in older adults involves addressing these age-related sleep challenges and implementing strategies to support restful sleep:

1. Maintain a Consistent Sleep Schedule:

- Encourage older adults to go to bed and wake up at the same times every day to regulate their circadian rhythms.

2. Create a Comfortable Sleep Environment:

- Ensure that the bedroom is conducive to sleep, with a comfortable mattress, appropriate bedding, and a dark, quiet atmosphere.

3. Limit Daytime Napping:

- While short naps can be refreshing, long daytime naps can interfere with nighttime sleep. Encourage shorter, strategic naps when needed.

4. Address Underlying Health Issues:

- Work with healthcare providers to manage chronic health conditions and address any medication-related sleep disturbances.

5. Promote Physical Activity:

- Encourage regular physical activity, which can improve sleep quality and overall health.

6. Manage Stress and Anxiety:

- Practice stress-reduction techniques, such as meditation, deep breathing, or progressive muscle relaxation.

7. Limit Stimulants and Alcohol:

- Reduce caffeine and alcohol intake, particularly in the hours leading up to bedtime.

8. Stay Socially Active:

- Encourage social engagement and activities to combat feelings of isolation and depression, which can affect sleep.

9. Seek Professional Help:

- If sleep problems persist, consult with a healthcare provider or sleep specialist to rule out underlying sleep disorders or other medical issues.

Understanding the unique sleep challenges faced by older adults and implementing strategies to address them is crucial for maintaining good sleep hygiene and overall well-being as we age. By prioritizing healthy sleep habits and seeking support when needed, older adults can enjoy restful and rejuvenating sleep in their later years.

Sleep and Aging: How It Affects Cognitive Function

As individuals grow older, sleep patterns change, and cognitive abilities may be influenced by these shifts. We'll discuss the impact of aging on cognitive function, how sleep plays a crucial role, and strategies to maintain cognitive health as we age.

Aging, Sleep, and Cognitive Function

Aging is associated with several changes in sleep patterns and cognitive function:

1. Changes in Sleep Architecture:

- **Reduced Deep Sleep:** Older adults often experience a decrease in deep, restorative sleep stages, such as slow-wave sleep (SWS), which plays a role in memory consolidation and cognitive function.
- **More Frequent Awakenings:** Aging can lead to more frequent awakenings during the night, reducing sleep continuity.

2. Cognitive Changes:

- **Memory:** Age-related cognitive changes can affect memory, including the ability to form new memories (encoding) and retrieve existing ones.
- **Executive Function:** Older adults may experience declines in executive functions, which include tasks such as planning, decision-

making, and multitasking.

- **Processing Speed:** Processing speed, or the ability to perform tasks quickly, may also decline with age.

3. Sleep Disorders:

- **Insomnia:** Insomnia becomes more common with age and can exacerbate cognitive difficulties.
- **Sleep Apnea:** The risk of sleep apnea increases with age and can lead to fragmented sleep and cognitive impairments.

4. Health Conditions:

- Chronic health conditions, such as diabetes, cardiovascular disease, and neurodegenerative disorders, can impact both sleep quality and cognitive function.

Maintaining Cognitive Health Through Sleep in Aging

Promoting cognitive health in older adults involves recognizing the impact of sleep on cognitive function and implementing strategies to support both:

1. Prioritize Sleep Quality:

- Emphasize the importance of maintaining good sleep hygiene practices, including consistent sleep schedules, a comfortable sleep environment, and stress reduction techniques.

2. Manage Sleep Disorders:

- Address sleep disorders, such as insomnia or sleep apnea, through consultation with healthcare providers or sleep specialists.

3. Engage in Cognitive Stimulation:

- Encourage activities that challenge the mind, such as puzzles, reading, learning a new language, or taking up a musical instrument.

4. Stay Physically Active:

- Regular physical activity can improve sleep quality and cognitive function. Encourage activities appropriate for individual fitness levels.

5. Maintain Social Connections:

- Social engagement and maintaining a supportive network can positively impact cognitive health.

6. Balanced Nutrition:

- Encourage a balanced diet rich in fruits, vegetables, whole grains, and healthy fats, as nutrition can influence both sleep quality and cognitive function.

7. Regular Health Checkups:

- Encourage regular health checkups to monitor and manage chronic health conditions that may impact sleep and cognitive function.

8. Cognitive Training Programs:

- Consider cognitive training programs designed to maintain and enhance cognitive abilities, especially if cognitive concerns arise.

Understanding the complex interplay between sleep and cognitive function in the context of aging is essential for promoting cognitive health in older adults. By prioritizing sleep quality, addressing sleep disorders, engaging in cognitive stimulation, and maintaining overall health and well-being, older adults can maximize their cognitive potential and enjoy a fulfilling and mentally vibrant later life.

Chapter 7: Strategies for Improving Sleep

Cognitive Behavioral Therapy for Insomnia (CBT-I)

Cognitive Behavioral Therapy for Insomnia (CBT-I). Insomnia is a common sleep disorder that can have a significant impact on one's quality of life, and CBT-I offers practical techniques and strategies to address it. We'll explore the principles of CBT-I, its components, and how it can help individuals improve their sleep patterns and overall well-being.

Understanding Insomnia

Insomnia is characterized by difficulty falling asleep, staying asleep, or waking up too early and not being able to return to sleep. It can lead to daytime fatigue, impaired cognitive function, mood disturbances, and decreased overall quality of life. Insomnia can be acute (short-term) or chronic (lasting for months or even years), and it often co-occurs with other medical or psychological conditions.

Cognitive Behavioral Therapy for Insomnia (CBT-I)

CBT-I is a structured, evidence-based approach to treating insomnia that targets the cognitive and behavioral factors contributing to sleep difficulties. It focuses on changing thought patterns and behaviors that perpetuate insomnia and aims to promote healthy sleep habits. Here are the key components of CBT-I:

1. Sleep Education:

- Understanding the science of sleep, sleep cycles, and the consequences of sleep deprivation is an essential foundation for CBT-I.

2. Sleep Restriction:

- This technique involves limiting the time spent in bed to match the actual amount of sleep obtained. It aims to consolidate sleep and reduce the time spent lying awake in bed.

3. Stimulus Control:

- Stimulus control techniques help individuals associate the bed and bedroom with sleep rather than wakefulness. This involves specific guidelines for what to do in the bedroom and what to avoid.

4. Sleep Hygiene:

- Sleep hygiene recommendations focus on creating a sleep-conducive environment, improving bedtime routines, and minimizing factors that can disrupt sleep.

5. Cognitive Restructuring:

- Cognitive restructuring involves identifying and challenging unhelpful thoughts and beliefs about sleep. This helps individuals reduce anxiety and frustration related to sleep.

6. Relaxation Techniques:

- Relaxation exercises, such as progressive muscle relaxation or deep breathing, can help reduce arousal and anxiety levels before bedtime.

7. Biofeedback and Mindfulness:

- Biofeedback and mindfulness techniques can enhance relaxation and awareness, promoting better sleep quality.

The Benefits of CBT-I

CBT-I has several advantages for individuals struggling with insomnia:

- **Long-Term Effectiveness:** CBT-I is associated with lasting improvements in sleep, making it a valuable alternative to medication for chronic insomnia.

- **Reduced Reliance on Medication:** CBT-I can help individuals reduce or eliminate the need for sleep medications, which can have side effects and the potential for dependency.
- **Improved Daytime Functioning:** Better sleep quality through CBT-I can lead to improved daytime alertness, mood, and cognitive performance.
- **Personalized Approach:** CBT-I is tailored to the individual, addressing their unique sleep patterns and concerns.
- **Minimal Side Effects:** Unlike some medications, CBT-I is associated with minimal side effects.

Seeking CBT-I

If you're struggling with insomnia, consider seeking a trained healthcare professional, such as a psychologist or sleep specialist, who can provide CBT-I. It typically involves several sessions and requires active participation from the individual.

CBT-I offers a holistic and effective approach to managing insomnia, addressing both the psychological and behavioral aspects of sleep difficulties. By implementing the principles and techniques of CBT-I, individuals can regain control over their sleep, improve sleep quality, and enhance their overall well-being.

Medications and Supplements for Sleep: Pros and Cons

While they can be effective in certain situations, it's essential to understand the potential benefits and risks associated with these sleep aids. We'll discuss common medications and supplements used for sleep, their pros and cons, and when they may be appropriate or should be approached with caution.

Medications for Sleep

Medications for sleep are typically prescribed for individuals with chronic insomnia or other sleep disorders when non-pharmacological interventions have not been successful. Here are some common types of sleep medications, along with their pros and cons:

1. Sedative-Hypnotics (e.g., Benzodiazepines and Non-Benzodiazepines):

Pros:

- **Short-Term Relief:** These medications can provide short-term relief for severe insomnia.
- **Rapid Onset:** They typically work quickly to help you fall asleep.

Cons:

- **Tolerance and Dependency:** Over time, individuals may develop tolerance and dependence on these medications, leading to a reduced effectiveness and withdrawal symptoms upon discontinuation.
- **Side Effects:** They can cause side effects like drowsiness, dizziness, and impaired coordination.
- **Memory and Cognitive Impairment:** Long-term use may lead to memory and cognitive impairments.

2. Melatonin Receptor Agonists:

Pros:

- **Minimal Dependency:** These medications have a lower risk of dependency compared to some other sleep medications.
- **Circadian Rhythm Regulation:** They can help regulate sleep-wake cycles and are often used for jet lag and shift work sleep disorder.

Cons:

- **Side Effects:** Side effects may include dizziness, headache, and next-day drowsiness.
- **Limited Effectiveness:** They may not be as effective for all types of insomnia.

3. Antidepressants (e.g., Trazodone and Doxepin):

Pros:

- **Dual Purpose:** Some antidepressants have sedative effects and can be useful for individuals with co-occurring depression or anxiety.

Cons:

- **Delayed Onset:** They may take several weeks to exert their full sleep-inducing effects.
- **Side Effects:** Antidepressants can have various side effects, including dry mouth, constipation, and weight gain.

Supplements for Sleep

Supplements for sleep are often used as over-the-counter alternatives to medications. While they are generally considered safer, they may not be as effective for severe or chronic sleep disturbances. Here are some common supplements used for sleep, along with their pros and cons:

1. Melatonin:

Pros:

- **Circadian Rhythm Regulation:** Melatonin supplements can help regulate sleep-wake cycles, making them useful for jet lag and shift work sleep disorder.
- **Minimal Side Effects:** They typically have few side effects.

Cons:

- **Variable Effectiveness:** Melatonin may not work for everyone, and the optimal dose can vary.

2. Valerian Root:

Pros:

- **Mild Sedative Effect:** Valerian root is believed to have a mild sedative effect and may help some individuals fall asleep.

Cons:

- **Variable Effectiveness:** Its effectiveness can vary widely from person to person.
- **Potential Interactions:** Valerian root may interact with other medications.

3. Magnesium:

Pros:

- **Muscle Relaxation:** Magnesium may help relax muscles and promote a sense of calm, aiding sleep.

Cons:

- **Effectiveness:** While magnesium can be beneficial for some, it may not address the underlying causes of insomnia in all cases.

4. L-Tryptophan:

Pros:

- **Precursor to Melatonin:** L-Tryptophan is a precursor to melatonin and serotonin, which are involved in sleep regulation.

Cons:

- **Mixed Research:** The evidence for its effectiveness in improving sleep is mixed.

Choosing the Right Approach

The use of medications and supplements for sleep should be approached with caution and, ideally, under the guidance of a healthcare professional. It's essential to weigh the potential benefits against the risks and consider alternative strategies for improving sleep, such as lifestyle changes and behavioral interventions. Medications and supplements may be appropriate in specific situations, but they should not be seen as the first-line treatment for insomnia or sleep disturbances. Understanding the pros and cons of these sleep aids can help individuals make informed decisions about their use.

Sleep Tracking and Monitoring Devices

We'll discuss the pros and cons of using these devices, their potential benefits, and considerations for those interested in integrating them into their sleep improvement strategies.

The Rise of Sleep Tracking Devices

In recent years, the market for sleep tracking and monitoring devices has grown significantly. These devices come in various forms, including wearable fitness trackers, smartwatches, and smartphone apps. They promise to provide valuable information about sleep duration, sleep stages, and sleep disturbances. Here's a closer look at the pros and cons of using sleep tracking devices:

Pros of Sleep Tracking Devices:

1. Awareness and Education:

- Sleep trackers can raise awareness about one's sleep patterns and habits, encouraging individuals to pay more attention to their sleep.

2. Objective Data:

- Sleep tracking devices offer objective data that can help individuals understand their sleep quality and identify potential issues.

3. Goal Setting:

- Many devices allow users to set sleep goals, promoting a sense of responsibility for their sleep health.

4. Sleep Trends:

- Over time, sleep data can reveal trends and patterns, aiding in the identification of sleep disorders or other issues.

5. Sleep Optimization:

- Armed with insights from sleep tracking, individuals can make informed decisions to optimize their sleep habits.

Cons of Sleep Tracking Devices:

1. Accuracy:

- The accuracy of sleep tracking devices can vary. Some may provide estimates rather than precise measurements of sleep stages.

2. Sleep Anxiety:

- Constant monitoring can lead to sleep-related anxiety or "orthosomnia," where individuals become overly concerned about achieving perfect sleep.

3. Disruption:

- The act of wearing a device or checking sleep data during the night can disrupt sleep and exacerbate sleep-related anxiety.

4. Limited Actionability:

- While sleep data can be informative, it may not always lead to actionable changes in sleep habits.

5. Privacy Concerns:

- Some individuals may have concerns about the privacy of their sleep data, especially when using smartphone apps or cloud-based services.

Considerations for Using Sleep Tracking Devices:

If you're considering using a sleep tracking device, here are some important considerations:

1. Choose a Reliable Device:

- Research and select a device with a reputation for accuracy in sleep tracking.

2. Balance Awareness and Obsession:

- Use sleep tracking as a tool for awareness and improvement rather than becoming obsessed with achieving perfect sleep.

3. Avoid Excessive Monitoring:

- Don't constantly check sleep data during the night, as this can disrupt sleep.

4. Focus on Patterns, Not Perfection:

- Pay attention to trends and patterns in your sleep data rather than striving for perfection.

5. Combine with Other Sleep Strategies:

- Use sleep tracking devices in conjunction with other sleep improvement strategies, such as good sleep hygiene practices and stress management.

Sleep Clinics and Professional Help

While many sleep issues can be managed with lifestyle changes, there are situations where seeking the expertise of healthcare professionals is crucial. We'll discuss the benefits of sleep clinics, the types of professionals involved in sleep medicine, and when it's advisable to seek professional help for sleep problems.

The Role of Sleep Clinics

Sleep clinics, also known as sleep centers or sleep disorder centers, are specialized facilities dedicated to diagnosing and treating sleep disorders. These clinics play a vital role in the field of sleep medicine and offer a range of services to individuals struggling with sleep-related issues. Here are some key aspects of sleep clinics:

1. Diagnosis of Sleep Disorders:

- Sleep clinics provide comprehensive evaluations and diagnostic testing to identify various sleep disorders, including sleep apnea, insomnia, narcolepsy, and restless legs syndrome.

2. Treatment and Management:

- Once a diagnosis is made, sleep clinics offer tailored treatment plans and strategies to manage sleep disorders effectively.

3. Polysomnography (Sleep Study):

- Sleep clinics often conduct polysomnography, a comprehensive sleep study that monitors various physiological parameters during sleep, including brain activity, eye movements, heart rate, and breathing.

4. Continuous Positive Airway Pressure (CPAP) Therapy:

- For individuals with sleep apnea, sleep clinics may prescribe and provide CPAP therapy, a highly effective treatment that uses a device to keep the airway open during sleep.

Types of Professionals in Sleep Medicine

Sleep medicine is a multidisciplinary field that involves various healthcare professionals with specialized training in diagnosing and treating sleep disorders. Some key professionals you may encounter in sleep clinics include:

1. Sleep Medicine Physicians:

- These medical doctors (MDs or DOs) specialize in sleep medicine and are experts in diagnosing and treating sleep disorders. They often oversee sleep clinic operations.

2. Respiratory Therapists:

- Respiratory therapists are trained to administer and educate patients about therapies such as CPAP for sleep apnea.

3. Sleep Technologists:

- Sleep technologists are responsible for conducting and monitoring sleep studies, ensuring accurate data collection during polysomnography.

4. Psychologists and Psychiatrists:

- Psychologists and psychiatrists with expertise in sleep may provide therapy for conditions like insomnia and contribute to the management of sleep-related mental health issues.

When to Seek Professional Help

While many individuals can improve their sleep through lifestyle changes and self-help strategies, there are situations where seeking professional help is advisable:

1. Persistent Sleep Problems:

- If sleep problems persist for several weeks and impact daily functioning, it's essential to consult a healthcare professional.

2. Suspected Sleep Disorders:

- If you suspect you have a sleep disorder, such as sleep apnea or restless legs syndrome, seeking professional evaluation is crucial.

3. Severe Symptoms:

- Severe symptoms such as loud snoring, choking or gasping during sleep, excessive daytime sleepiness, or frequent nighttime awakenings should prompt a visit to a sleep clinic.

4. Ineffectiveness of Self-Help Strategies:

- If self-help strategies and lifestyle changes do not improve sleep quality or symptoms worsen, professional evaluation is warranted.

5. Co-Occurring Medical Conditions:

- Individuals with underlying medical conditions, such as heart disease, diabetes, or obesity, may benefit from a sleep evaluation as sleep disorders can exacerbate these conditions.

Lifestyle Changes for Sustainable Sleep Improvement

While there are various strategies and interventions available for better sleep, focusing on lifestyle modifications can have a lasting and positive impact on your sleep patterns. We'll discuss key lifestyle changes that can promote healthy sleep and enhance overall well-being.

The Importance of Lifestyle in Sleep Health

Lifestyle factors play a significant role in determining the quality and duration of your sleep. By making informed choices and adopting healthy habits, you can create an environment that supports restorative sleep. Here are key lifestyle changes to consider:

1. Consistent Sleep Schedule:

- Go to bed and wake up at the same times every day, even on weekends. Consistency helps regulate your body's internal clock.

2. Create a Relaxing Bedtime Routine:

- Establish a calming bedtime routine to signal to your body that it's time to wind down. This could include activities like reading, gentle stretching, or practicing relaxation techniques.

3. Optimize Your Sleep Environment:

- Ensure that your bedroom is conducive to sleep. Keep it dark, quiet, and at a comfortable temperature. Invest in a comfortable mattress and pillows.

4. Limit Exposure to Screens Before Bed:

- The blue light emitted by smartphones, tablets, and computers can interfere with your body's production of melatonin, a hormone that regulates sleep. Limit screen time at least an hour before bedtime.

5. Manage Stress and Anxiety:

- Stress and anxiety can disrupt sleep. Engage in stress-reduction techniques such as meditation, deep breathing, or mindfulness to calm your mind before sleep.

6. Regular Physical Activity:

- Regular exercise can improve sleep quality. Aim for at least 30 minutes of moderate exercise most days of the week, but avoid vigorous exercise close to bedtime.

7. Watch Your Diet:

- Avoid heavy, spicy, or large meals close to bedtime. Caffeine and nicotine are stimulants that can interfere with sleep, so limit their consumption, especially in the evening.

8. Be Mindful of Alcohol:

- While alcohol may initially make you feel drowsy, it can disrupt sleep patterns and lead to fragmented sleep. Limit alcohol intake, especially before bedtime.

9. Manage Daylight Exposure:

- Exposure to natural light during the day can help regulate your circadian rhythms. Spend time outdoors, especially in the morning.

10. Limit Naps:

- While short daytime naps can be refreshing, long or irregular napping can interfere with nighttime sleep. If you need to nap, keep it short (20-30 minutes).

11. Monitor Your Sleep:

- Consider keeping a sleep diary to track your sleep patterns and identify areas for improvement.

12. Mindful Consumption of Sleep Aids:

- If you use sleep aids or supplements, do so under the guidance of a healthcare professional and for a limited time. Relying on them long-term can have negative consequences.

13. Seek Professional Help When Needed:

- If lifestyle changes and self-help strategies do not lead to improvements in your sleep quality, consider consulting a healthcare professional or sleep specialist.

Chapter 8: The Consequences of Sleep Deprivation

Cognitive Impairment and Memory Problems

Sleep plays a crucial role in cognitive function, and when it's consistently lacking, it can lead to a range of cognitive difficulties. We'll delve into the impact of sleep deprivation on cognitive abilities, memory formation, and strategies for mitigating these effects.

The Connection Between Sleep and Cognitive Function

Sleep is essential for various cognitive functions, including memory consolidation, attention, problem-solving, and decision-making. When we don't get enough sleep, our cognitive abilities are compromised. Here's how sleep deprivation affects cognition:

1. Memory Problems:

- Sleep is crucial for memory consolidation, the process by which new information is transferred from short-term memory to long-term memory. Sleep-deprived individuals often struggle with both short-term and long-term memory.

2. Attention and Concentration:

- Sleep deprivation impairs sustained attention and the ability to focus on tasks, leading to decreased productivity and increased errors.

3. Problem-Solving and Creativity:

- Sleep-deprived individuals may have difficulty solving complex problems and thinking creatively. Sleep is thought to enhance insight and problem-solving abilities.

4. Decision-Making:

- Sleep loss can lead to poor decision-making and impulsivity, as it affects the brain's prefrontal cortex, which is responsible for executive functions.

5. Reaction Time:

- Sleep deprivation can slow reaction times, making activities like driving or operating machinery dangerous.

The Impact of Sleep Deprivation on Memory

Memory impairment is a well-documented consequence of sleep deprivation. Here's how sleep loss affects different types of memory:

1. Short-Term Memory:

- Sleep-deprived individuals often struggle with short-term memory, making it challenging to remember recent events or information.

2. Long-Term Memory:

- Sleep plays a critical role in transferring information from short-term memory to long-term memory. Without sufficient sleep, this process is disrupted, leading to difficulties in retaining and recalling information over time.

3. Emotional Memory:

- Sleep deprivation can intensify the emotional components of memory, making negative experiences more emotionally charged.

4. Procedural Memory:

- Procedural memory, which involves skills and habits, can also be negatively affected by sleep loss. Tasks that require precision and consistency may suffer.

Strategies for Mitigating Cognitive Impairment Due to Sleep Deprivation

While the best way to mitigate the cognitive effects of sleep deprivation is to prioritize and consistently obtain adequate sleep, there are strategies to help manage the consequences:

1. Prioritize Sleep: Make sleep a priority by setting a regular sleep schedule and ensuring you get the recommended 7-9 hours of sleep per night.

2. Create a Sleep-Conducive Environment: Make your bedroom comfortable, quiet, and dark to optimize sleep quality.

3. Limit Caffeine and Alcohol: Avoid caffeine and alcohol in the hours leading up to bedtime, as they can interfere with sleep.

4. Manage Stress: Practice stress-reduction techniques, such as mindfulness, meditation, or progressive muscle relaxation, to calm the mind before sleep.

5. Naps: Short, strategic naps (20-30 minutes) can help mitigate some of the cognitive effects of sleep deprivation.

6. Seek Professional Help: If sleep deprivation persists despite your efforts, consult with a healthcare professional or sleep specialist to identify underlying sleep disorders and receive appropriate treatment.

The Relationship Between Sleep Deprivation and Accidents

Sleep plays an essential role in maintaining alertness and cognitive function, and when it's lacking, the risk of accidents, both on the road and in the workplace, significantly increases. We'll delve into the impact of sleep deprivation on accident risk, the industries and situations most affected, and strategies for preventing accidents related to inadequate sleep.

Understanding the Sleep-Related Accident Risk

Sleep deprivation poses a considerable risk to safety, leading to an increased likelihood of accidents and errors in various settings. Here's an overview of how sleep deprivation contributes to accidents:

1. Impaired Cognitive Function:

- Sleep deprivation impairs cognitive function, including attention, reaction time, and decision-making. This can lead to errors, accidents, and decreased situational awareness.

2. Microsleeps:

- In severe cases of sleep deprivation, individuals may experience "microsleeps," brief episodes of sleep that last for a few seconds. During a microsleep, individuals are effectively asleep, even if their eyes are open, which can be especially dangerous while driving or operating machinery.

3. Increased Risk-Taking Behavior:

- Sleep-deprived individuals are more likely to engage in risky behaviors, including taking chances and making impulsive decisions.

4. Decreased Alertness:

- Prolonged wakefulness reduces alertness, making individuals more prone to lapses in attention and reduced awareness of their surroundings.

Industries Most Affected by Sleep-Related Accidents

While sleep-related accidents can occur in any industry or setting, certain sectors are particularly vulnerable due to the nature of their work and schedules. These industries include:

1. Transportation:

- The transportation industry, including trucking, aviation, and maritime, is highly affected by sleep-related accidents. Fatigue-related accidents among truck drivers, for example, are a significant concern.

2. Healthcare:

- Healthcare professionals, especially those working extended shifts, are at risk of making errors due to sleep deprivation, which can jeopardize patient safety.

3. Manufacturing and Construction:

- Workers in these industries may operate heavy machinery or perform tasks that require precision, making sleep-deprivation-related accidents a significant concern.

4. Emergency Services:

- Firefighters, police officers, and paramedics often work irregular hours and may experience sleep deprivation, impacting their ability to respond effectively in emergency situations.

Preventing Sleep-Related Accidents

Preventing accidents related to sleep deprivation requires a combination of individual and organizational efforts:

1. Prioritize Sleep: Individuals should prioritize getting adequate and quality sleep by maintaining a consistent sleep schedule and ensuring a sleep-conducive environment.

2. Limit Shift Duration: Organizations should implement policies that limit the duration of extended shifts and promote regular breaks for employees.

3. Promote Education: Both individuals and employers should educate themselves and their teams about the risks of sleep deprivation and the importance of sleep hygiene.

4. Encourage Napping: In industries with irregular schedules, organizations can provide designated spaces for short naps during breaks.

5. Use Technology: In transportation, technology such as fatigue monitoring systems can help identify signs of sleepiness and alert drivers or operators to take breaks.

6. Seek Help for Sleep Disorders: Individuals with sleep disorders should seek medical evaluation and treatment to address underlying issues.

Sleep Deprivation and Workplace Productivity

Sleep is closely linked to cognitive function, concentration, and overall performance, and when it's compromised, it can have detrimental effects on an individual's ability to work efficiently and effectively. We'll delve into how sleep deprivation affects workplace productivity, strategies for managing sleep-related productivity issues, and the role of employers in promoting healthy sleep habits among their employees.

The Impact of Sleep Deprivation on Workplace Productivity

Sleep deprivation can have profound negative effects on an individual's ability to perform effectively in the workplace. Here are some key ways in which inadequate sleep can impact productivity:

1. Decreased Cognitive Function:

- Sleep deprivation impairs cognitive functions such as memory, attention, problem-solving, and decision-making. This can result in reduced efficiency and an increased likelihood of making mistakes.

2. Reduced Concentration:

- Individuals who are sleep-deprived often struggle to maintain focus and concentration, leading to difficulty completing tasks and increased procrastination.

3. Slower Reaction Times:

- Sleep-deprived individuals may have slower reaction times, which can be especially problematic in jobs that require quick responses or operating machinery.

4. Increased Errors:

- The likelihood of errors and accidents at work significantly rises when employees are sleep-deprived. This can have serious consequences, particularly in safety-sensitive industries.

5. Impaired Communication:

- Sleep deprivation can affect verbal and non-verbal communication, leading to misunderstandings and breakdowns in teamwork.

6. Decreased Creativity:

- Sleep is essential for creative thinking and problem-solving. Lack of sleep can stifle innovation and hinder the generation of new ideas.

7. Higher Absenteeism:

- Sleep-deprived employees are more likely to take sick days or absenteeism due to health issues related to inadequate sleep.

Strategies for Managing Sleep-Related Productivity Issues

Individuals and employers can take steps to manage and mitigate sleep-related productivity issues in the workplace:

For Individuals:

1. Prioritize Sleep: Make sleep a priority and aim for 7-9 hours of quality sleep each night.

2. Create a Consistent Sleep Schedule: Go to bed and wake up at the same times every day, even on weekends, to regulate your body's internal clock.

3. Establish a Bedtime Routine: Develop a calming pre-sleep routine to signal to your body that it's time to wind down.

4. Optimize Your Sleep Environment: Make sure your bedroom is comfortable, quiet, and dark to enhance sleep quality.

5. Limit Screen Time: Avoid screens (phones, tablets, computers) at least an hour before bedtime to reduce exposure to blue light that can disrupt sleep.

6. Manage Stress: Practice stress-reduction techniques, such as meditation or deep breathing exercises, to calm your mind before sleep.

For Employers:

1. Promote a Culture of Well-being: Encourage and support healthy sleep habits among employees by promoting the importance of sleep for productivity and well-being.

2. Flexible Schedules: Consider offering flexible work schedules that allow employees to better align their work hours with their natural sleep patterns.

3. Breaks and Nap Opportunities: Provide designated spaces for short naps during breaks, especially for employees working long shifts.

4. Education and Training: Offer educational resources and training programs on sleep hygiene and time management to help employees manage their sleep and workload effectively.

5. Employee Assistance Programs (EAPs): Include sleep-related resources in EAPs to provide support for employees facing sleep difficulties.

Sleep and Relationships: How It Impacts Interpersonal Dynamics

Sleep plays a crucial role in emotional regulation, communication, and overall well-being, and when it's compromised, it can strain relationships. We'll delve into the ways in which sleep deprivation can impact relationships, strategies for maintaining healthy relationships despite sleep-related challenges, and the importance of communication and mutual support.

The Impact of Sleep Deprivation on Relationships

Sleep deprivation can have far-reaching effects on personal relationships, including those with partners, family members, and friends. Here are some key ways in which inadequate sleep can impact relationships:

1. Increased Irritability and Conflict:

- Sleep-deprived individuals are more likely to be irritable and quick to anger, leading to conflicts and arguments within relationships.

2. Reduced Empathy and Understanding:

- Sleep deprivation can impair the ability to understand and empathize with others, making it challenging to provide emotional support.

3. Communication Breakdown:

- Poor sleep can lead to miscommunication, misunderstandings, and a breakdown in effective communication between partners or within families.

4. Emotional Distance:

- Chronic sleep deprivation can create emotional distance between individuals, as they may be less inclined to engage in social activities or spend quality time together.

5. Decreased Libido:

- Sleep deprivation can negatively impact sexual desire and performance, potentially affecting intimate relationships.

6. Negative Mood:

- Sleep-deprived individuals are more likely to experience negative moods, which can cast a shadow over social interactions and relationships.

7. Increased Stress:

- Sleep deprivation can contribute to overall stress levels, making it difficult to handle relationship challenges effectively.

Strategies for Maintaining Healthy Relationships Despite Sleep-Related Challenges

Despite the challenges posed by sleep deprivation, individuals can take steps to maintain healthy relationships:

1. Open Communication: Discuss sleep-related issues with your partner or loved ones. Let them know how sleep deprivation may be affecting your mood and behavior.

2. Mutual Support: Partners and family members can support each other in getting adequate sleep. This may involve sharing childcare responsibilities or household chores to free up time for rest.

3. Sleep Synchronization: Try to synchronize sleep schedules with your partner as much as possible to ensure you both get the rest you need.

4. Conflict Resolution: When conflicts arise due to sleep-related irritability, address them calmly and constructively. Consider seeking the help of a relationship counselor if necessary.

5. Self-Care: Prioritize self-care and sleep hygiene to improve your sleep quality. This can have positive ripple effects on your mood and relationships.

6. Seek Professional Help: If sleep issues persist and significantly impact your relationships, consider seeking guidance from a sleep specialist or therapist.

Long-Term Health Consequences of Chronic Sleep Deprivation

In this final chapter, we delve into the long-term health consequences of chronic sleep deprivation. While the immediate effects of inadequate sleep are concerning, the cumulative impact over months and years can be even more detrimental. We'll explore how chronic sleep deprivation can affect various aspects of physical and mental health, strategies for mitigating these long-term effects, and the importance of prioritizing sleep for overall well-being.

The Accumulative Toll of Chronic Sleep Deprivation

Chronic sleep deprivation, defined as consistently not getting enough sleep over an extended period, can have severe consequences for overall health. Here's how inadequate sleep can impact long-term well-being:

1. Cardiovascular Health:

- Chronic sleep deprivation is linked to an increased risk of hypertension (high blood pressure), heart disease, and stroke. It can also disrupt the body's regulation of stress hormones, further impacting heart health.

2. Metabolic Health:

- Long-term sleep deprivation is associated with insulin resistance, obesity, and an increased risk of type 2 diabetes. Poor sleep can disrupt the body's regulation of glucose and appetite hormones.

3. Immune Function:

- Inadequate sleep weakens the immune system, making individuals more susceptible to infections and chronic inflammation. This can contribute to various health conditions.

4. Mental Health:

- Chronic sleep deprivation is closely linked to mental health disorders such as depression and anxiety. It can exacerbate existing mental health conditions and contribute to their onset.

5. Cognitive Decline:

- Over time, inadequate sleep can lead to cognitive decline and an increased risk of neurodegenerative diseases like Alzheimer's and dementia.

6. Reduced Life Expectancy:

- Numerous studies have suggested that chronic sleep deprivation is associated with a higher risk of mortality and reduced life expectancy.

Mitigating the Long-Term Effects of Chronic Sleep Deprivation

While the long-term health consequences of chronic sleep deprivation are concerning, individuals can take steps to mitigate these effects:

1. Prioritize Sleep: Make sleep a non-negotiable priority in your life. Aim for 7-9 hours of quality sleep each night.

2. Consistent Sleep Schedule: Maintain a consistent sleep schedule, even on weekends, to regulate your body's internal clock.

3. Create a Sleep-Friendly Environment: Ensure your bedroom is conducive to sleep, with a comfortable mattress, pillows, and a dark, quiet atmosphere.

4. Practice Good Sleep Hygiene: Adopt healthy sleep habits, such as limiting screen time before bed, avoiding caffeine and alcohol close to bedtime, and managing stress.

5. Regular Physical Activity: Engage in regular exercise, as it can improve sleep quality and overall health.

6. Seek Professional Help: If you have chronic sleep issues or suspect a sleep disorder, consult with a healthcare professional or sleep specialist for evaluation and treatment.

Chapter 9: Sleep and Dreams

The Science of Dreams: What Do They Mean?

Dreams have captivated human curiosity for centuries, and while they remain enigmatic in many ways, scientific research has shed light on their functions, mechanisms, and potential significance.

The Nature of Dreams

Dreams are a mysterious realm of human experience that occur during rapid eye movement (REM) sleep, a stage characterized by heightened brain activity and vivid mental imagery. While the content of dreams can vary widely from person to person, there are common themes, emotions, and symbols that often recur in dream experiences.

The Function of Dreams

Researchers have proposed several theories about the function of dreams:

1. Memory Consolidation: Some theories suggest that dreams play a role in consolidating and organizing memories, helping us process and make sense of the events and information encountered during waking hours.

2. Emotional Processing: Dreams can serve as a means of processing and regulating emotions, providing a safe space to explore and confront emotional challenges.

3. Problem-Solving: Dreams have been credited with aiding problem-solving and creative thinking by presenting novel solutions or perspectives on waking-life issues.

4. Processing Unconscious Material: Psychologists like Sigmund Freud proposed that dreams serve as a gateway to the unconscious mind, allowing suppressed thoughts and desires to surface.

5. Evolutionary Theories: Some theories posit that dreaming may have evolved as a way to rehearse and prepare for real-life threats or challenges, contributing to survival and adaptation.

Interpreting Dreams

Dream interpretation has a long history, from ancient civilizations to modern psychoanalysis. While there is no definitive method for interpreting dreams, individuals often find personal meaning in their dreams based on their unique life experiences, emotions, and beliefs.

The Role of Culture and Personal Experience:

- Cultural and personal factors heavily influence dream symbolism and interpretation. What a dream symbolizes to one person may differ significantly from another's interpretation.

Modern Approaches:

- Some psychologists use therapeutic techniques like dream analysis to explore the emotional and psychological content of dreams, helping individuals gain insights into their feelings and behaviors.

Lucid Dreaming:

- Lucid dreaming is a state in which the dreamer is aware they are dreaming and can sometimes exert control over the dream's narrative. This state offers opportunities for self-exploration and creativity.

Nightmares and Night Terrors:

- Nightmares are distressing dreams that often involve fear or anxiety, while night terrors are characterized by sudden awakenings with intense fear and confusion. These experiences can provide insights into unresolved traumas or anxieties.

The Unconscious Mind:

- Dreams may offer glimpses into the workings of the unconscious mind, revealing aspects of our inner world that are not readily apparent in waking life.

Lucid Dreaming: Controlling Your Dreams

Lucid dreaming offers a unique and immersive experience within the realm of dreams and has fascinated psychologists, researchers, and dream enthusiasts for decades. We'll explore what lucid dreaming is, how it works, techniques for inducing lucidity, and the potential benefits and applications of this extraordinary state of consciousness.

Understanding Lucid Dreaming

Lucid dreaming is a state in which the dreamer is aware that they are dreaming while still immersed in the dream itself. This awareness can range from a subtle realization that "this is a dream" to full control over the dream's content, where the dreamer can manipulate the dream world at will. Lucid dreams often feel incredibly vivid and real, blurring the line between dream and waking reality.

The Experience of Lucid Dreaming

Lucid dreams offer a wide range of experiences and possibilities:

1. Control: In a lucid dream, the dreamer may gain the ability to control elements of the dream, such as flying, changing the environment, or interacting with dream characters.

2. Exploration: Lucid dreamers can explore surreal and fantastical landscapes, meet imaginary creatures, or visit places from their past.

3. Creativity: Lucid dreaming provides a fertile ground for creative inspiration, as dreamers can actively engage with their subconscious mind and generate innovative ideas.

4. Overcoming Nightmares: Lucid dreaming techniques can be used to confront and transform nightmares into more positive dream experiences.

Techniques for Inducing Lucid Dreams

Lucid dreaming can be cultivated through various techniques:

1. Reality Checks: Lucid dreamers often perform reality checks throughout the day, asking themselves whether they are dreaming or awake. This habit can carry over into dreams, leading to lucidity when a dreamer realizes something unusual.

2. Dream Journals: Keeping a dream journal encourages dream recall and recognition of recurring dream signs or patterns, increasing the likelihood of becoming lucid.

3. Mnemonic Induction of Lucid Dreams (MILD): This technique involves setting the intention to become lucid before falling asleep, often combined with visualizing a recent dream.

4. Wake-Back-to-Bed (WBTB): WBTB involves waking up during the night, staying awake for a brief period, and then returning to sleep with the intention of entering a lucid dream state.

5. Wake-Initiated Lucid Dreams (WILD): In WILD, the dreamer attempts to maintain awareness as they transition from wakefulness to a dream state during the onset of sleep.

Potential Benefits of Lucid Dreaming

Lucid dreaming isn't just a captivating experience; it also has potential practical applications:

1. Overcoming Fears: Lucid dreaming can be used as a tool to confront and overcome fears or phobias in a safe dream environment.

2. Creative Problem Solving: Lucid dreams can inspire creative solutions to real-life problems by engaging with the subconscious mind.

3. Enhancing Skills: Some individuals use lucid dreaming to practice skills or rehearse scenarios, such as public speaking or sports.

4. Personal Growth: Lucid dreaming can facilitate self-discovery, exploration of one's psyche, and personal growth.

Nightmares and Night Terrors: Causes and Coping Strategies

Nightmares are distressing dreams that evoke fear, anxiety, or sadness and are often vividly remembered upon waking. Night terrors, on the other hand, are episodes of intense fear or panic during sleep, typically accompanied by physical symptoms and sometimes even sleepwalking. We'll delve into the causes of nightmares and night terrors, their impact on well-being, and strategies for coping with and preventing these disruptive nocturnal occurrences.

Understanding Nightmares and Night Terrors

Nightmares:

Nightmares are vivid and distressing dreams that can evoke strong emotions such as fear, anxiety, sadness, or anger. They often wake the dreamer, leaving them with clear and detailed memories of the dream content. Nightmares typically occur during rapid eye movement (REM) sleep, which is the stage of sleep associated with heightened brain activity and intense dreaming.

Night Terrors:

Night terrors, also known as sleep terrors, are sudden episodes of extreme fear, panic, or terror that occur during non-REM (NREM) sleep, usually within the first few hours of falling asleep. Unlike nightmares, individuals experiencing night terrors are often unresponsive and may exhibit physical symptoms such as rapid breathing, increased heart rate, and even sleepwalking.

Causes of Nightmares and Night Terrors

Both nightmares and night terrors can have multiple causes, including:

1. Stress and Anxiety: High levels of stress or anxiety can contribute to the occurrence of nightmares and night terrors.

2. Trauma and PTSD: Individuals who have experienced trauma, including post-traumatic stress disorder (PTSD), are more prone to nightmares and night terrors.

3. Medications: Certain medications, including antidepressants and sleep aids, can trigger vivid dreams and nightmares as side effects.

4. Sleep Disorders: Sleep disorders such as sleep apnea and restless legs syndrome may increase the likelihood of night terrors.

5. Fever or Illness: Night terrors can be more common in children when they have a fever or illness.

Coping Strategies for Nightmares and Night Terrors

1. Stress Reduction: Practicing stress-reduction techniques, such as mindfulness, meditation, and deep breathing exercises, can help reduce the frequency and intensity of nightmares and night terrors.

2. Establish a Relaxing Bedtime Routine: Create a calming bedtime routine to signal to your body that it's time to wind down and prepare for sleep.

3. Maintain a Consistent Sleep Schedule: Going to bed and waking up at the same times each day can help regulate your sleep patterns and reduce the occurrence of night terrors.

4. Create a Comfortable Sleep Environment: Ensure your bedroom is conducive to sleep, with a comfortable mattress, cozy bedding, and a dark, quiet atmosphere.

5. Medication Review: If nightmares are linked to medication use, consult your healthcare provider to discuss potential alternative medications or adjustments to your current treatment plan.

6. Address Underlying Conditions: If you suspect an underlying sleep disorder or mental health condition is contributing to nightmares or night terrors, seek professional evaluation and treatment.

7. Safety Precautions: If night terrors involve sleepwalking or other potentially dangerous behaviors, take safety precautions such as installing gates or locks to prevent injury.

Sleep Disorders Related to Dreams: REM Sleep Behavior Disorder

RBD is a fascinating yet potentially disruptive condition in which individuals physically act out their dreams during REM sleep, often leading to vivid and sometimes dangerous dream enactments. We'll delve into the causes, symptoms, diagnosis, and management of RBD, shedding light on this unique sleep disorder and its impact on those who experience it.

Understanding REM Sleep Behavior Disorder (RBD)

REM Sleep Behavior Disorder is a sleep disorder characterized by the loss of normal muscle atonia during REM sleep. Normally, during REM sleep, a state associated with vivid dreaming, the brain sends signals to inhibit muscle activity to prevent physical movements corresponding to dream actions. In RBD, this mechanism malfunctions, allowing individuals to physically act out their dreams, sometimes to an extreme degree.

Symptoms of REM Sleep Behavior Disorder

The hallmark symptom of RBD is the physical enactment of dreams during REM sleep. This can manifest as:

1. Vocalizations: Individuals may shout, scream, or speak during dream enactment.

2. Motor Movements: Complex motor behaviors such as punching, kicking, or flailing limbs can occur during REM sleep.

3. Thrashing: Some individuals may thrash around in bed, often violently.

4. Falling or Jumping Out of Bed: In severe cases, individuals may even jump or fall out of bed while dreaming.

5. Injury: RBD can lead to injuries to the affected individual or their sleep partner.

Causes and Risk Factors of RBD

The exact causes of RBD are not fully understood, but several factors may contribute:

1. Neurodegenerative Conditions: RBD can be associated with neurodegenerative disorders such as Parkinson's disease and multiple system atrophy.

2. Medications: Some medications, particularly certain antidepressants and antipsychotics, have been linked to the development of RBD.

3. Idiopathic RBD: In some cases, RBD occurs without an identifiable underlying cause, referred to as idiopathic RBD.

Diagnosis and Management of RBD

Diagnosing RBD typically involves a combination of clinical evaluation and sleep studies, including polysomnography. Treatment and management strategies include:

1. Medication: Clonazepam, a medication that suppresses REM sleep-related muscle activity, is often prescribed to reduce symptoms and prevent injury.

2. Safety Measures: Creating a safe sleep environment, such as removing sharp objects from the bedroom and installing bed rails, can help prevent injuries during dream enactment.

3. Lifestyle Changes: Avoiding alcohol and certain medications that can exacerbate RBD symptoms may be recommended.

4. Regular Follow-Up: Individuals with RBD, especially those with an underlying neurodegenerative condition, may require regular follow-up with a healthcare provider to monitor their condition.

The Role of Dreams in Mental Health

Dreams have long been a subject of fascination for psychologists and researchers, as they provide a unique window into the subconscious mind. We'll delve into how dreams can impact mental well-being, the ways in which they may reflect or influence emotional states, and their role in the diagnosis and treatment of mental health disorders.

The Influence of Dreams on Mental Health

Dreams play a complex role in mental health, and their impact can vary significantly from person to person. Here are some ways in which dreams are intertwined with mental well-being:

1. Emotional Processing:

- Dreams can serve as a tool for processing and regulating emotions. They provide a safe space for the mind to explore and confront difficult emotions, experiences, and unresolved issues.

2. Reflection of Emotional States:

- The emotional content of dreams often mirrors an individual's waking emotional states. Stress, anxiety, depression, and joy can all manifest in dream narratives.

3. Trauma and PTSD:

- For individuals who have experienced trauma, dreams may replay traumatic events. These dreams can be distressing but also offer opportunities for processing and healing.

4. Creative Problem Solving:

- Dreams have been credited with aiding creative problem solving. Innovators and artists throughout history have drawn inspiration from their dreams.

5. Sleep Disorders and Mental Health:

- Sleep disorders, such as insomnia or nightmares, can exacerbate mental health conditions or even contribute to their development.

Dreams in Mental Health Diagnosis and Treatment

1. Dream Analysis:

- Some therapeutic approaches, such as Jungian or Freudian psychoanalysis, involve dream analysis to gain insights into an individual's unconscious mind and emotional conflicts.

2. Post-Traumatic Stress Disorder (PTSD):

- Nightmares related to traumatic experiences are a common symptom of PTSD. Treatment approaches, such as exposure therapy, may target these nightmares to alleviate symptoms.

3. Substance Abuse and Recovery:

- Dreams can play a role in addiction and recovery. Some individuals in recovery report vivid dreams related to substance use, while others find solace and inspiration in their dreams as they work towards sobriety.

4. Depression and Anxiety:

- Disturbed sleep patterns and vivid, emotionally charged dreams are associated with mood disorders like depression and anxiety. Addressing sleep quality is often a crucial component of treatment.

5. Mindfulness and Dream Yoga:

- Mindfulness practices, including dream yoga in some spiritual traditions, encourage awareness and presence in the dream state. These practices may promote self-awareness and emotional regulation.

Chapter 10: Finding Balance

Prioritizing Sleep in a Busy World

In this final chapter, we address the challenge of prioritizing sleep in a fast-paced and demanding world. Despite the well-established importance of sleep for overall health and well-being, many individuals struggle to make it a priority in their lives. We'll explore the barriers to adequate sleep, the consequences of neglecting it, and practical strategies for finding balance and making sleep a non-negotiable aspect of self-care.

The Sleep-Deprived World

In today's modern society, sleep often takes a back seat to other demands, such as work, social commitments, and digital distractions. Common barriers to prioritizing sleep include:

1. Work Demands: Long working hours, irregular schedules, and the expectation of constant connectivity can interfere with sleep.

2. Social Pressure: Social activities, entertainment, and the desire to be "always on" can lead to late nights and reduced sleep.

3. Screen Time: The use of screens, especially before bedtime, can disrupt sleep patterns by interfering with the body's natural circadian rhythms.

4. Stress and Anxiety: High levels of stress and anxiety can make it difficult to relax and fall asleep, perpetuating a cycle of sleep deprivation.

The Consequences of Sleep Neglect

Neglecting sleep can have profound consequences for physical, mental, and emotional well-being. These consequences include:

1. Cognitive Impairment: Sleep deprivation impairs cognitive functions such as memory, decision-making, and problem-solving.

2. Mood Disturbances: Insufficient sleep can lead to mood swings, irritability, and an increased risk of mental health disorders.

3. Health Risks: Chronic sleep deprivation is associated with a higher risk of chronic diseases such as heart disease, diabetes, and obesity.

4. Reduced Productivity: Sleep-deprived individuals are less productive and efficient at work, ultimately affecting their professional success.

5. Strained Relationships: Sleep deprivation can lead to irritability and conflict in relationships, affecting both personal and professional connections.

Strategies for Prioritizing Sleep

Despite the challenges of modern life, there are practical strategies for making sleep a priority:

1. Set Boundaries: Establish boundaries for work and social commitments to ensure you have dedicated time for sleep.

2. Create a Bedtime Routine: Develop a calming bedtime routine that signals to your body that it's time to wind down.

3. Practice Good Sleep Hygiene: Adopt healthy sleep habits, such as avoiding screens before bed and keeping your sleep environment comfortable.

4. Manage Stress: Explore stress-reduction techniques such as mindfulness, meditation, and yoga to manage stress and anxiety.

5. Communicate: Discuss the importance of sleep with family members, friends, and colleagues to gain their support and understanding.

6. Prioritize Self-Care: Recognize that adequate sleep is a form of self-care, and prioritize it as you would nutrition, exercise, and mental well-being.

Combating Sleep Myths and Misconceptions

Dispelling these myths and understanding the science of sleep can empower individuals to make informed decisions about their sleep habits and overall well-being. We'll address common misunderstandings about sleep duration, quality, and the factors that influence our sleep patterns.

Myth 1: "I Can Get By on Just a Few Hours of Sleep"

One of the most damaging myths is the belief that some people can thrive on minimal sleep. In reality, most adults require 7-9 hours of quality sleep per night for optimal health and functioning. Chronic sleep deprivation can have severe consequences for physical and mental well-being.

Myth 2: "Sleeping In on Weekends Can Compensate for Lost Sleep During the Week"

While catching up on sleep over the weekend can provide temporary relief, it doesn't fully compensate for chronic sleep deprivation. Irregular sleep patterns disrupt the body's circadian rhythms and can lead to long-term health issues.

Myth 3: "Alcohol and Sleep Medications Improve Sleep"

While alcohol and sleep medications may initially induce drowsiness, they often lead to disrupted sleep patterns, reduced sleep quality, and dependence. These substances can exacerbate sleep problems rather than solve them.

Myth 4: "I Can Function Normally with Insomnia"

Insomnia is not a normal or sustainable state of being. Prolonged insomnia can lead to cognitive impairment, mood disturbances, and increased risk of chronic diseases. Seeking treatment for insomnia is essential for overall well-being.

Myth 5: "Snoring Is Harmless"

While occasional snoring is common, chronic and loud snoring can be a sign of sleep apnea, a potentially serious sleep disorder that affects breathing during sleep. Sleep apnea can have significant health consequences and should not be ignored.

Myth 6: "Watching TV or Using Screens Helps Me Relax Before Bed"

Screens emit blue light, which suppresses the production of melatonin, a hormone that regulates sleep. Engaging with screens before bedtime can disrupt sleep patterns by delaying the onset of sleep.

Myth 7: "A Warm Glass of Milk Will Help Me Fall Asleep"

While warm milk contains the amino acid tryptophan, which is a precursor to melatonin, the effect is minimal. A balanced diet and healthy sleep habits are more effective for promoting quality sleep.

Myth 8: "Napping Is for the Lazy"

Napping can be a healthy and restorative practice when done strategically. Short power naps (around 20-30 minutes) can boost alertness and productivity. However, excessively long or late-day naps can interfere with nighttime sleep.

The Connection Between Sleep and Overall Well-being

In this final chapter, we bring together all the insights and knowledge we've explored in this book to underscore the profound connection between sleep and overall well-being. Sleep is not an isolated aspect of our lives; it is an essential foundation for physical, mental, and emotional health. We'll revisit key takeaways and provide a comprehensive perspective on how prioritizing sleep can lead to a happier, healthier, and more fulfilling life.

The Sleep-Well-being Nexus

The intricate relationship between sleep and overall well-being can be summarized as follows:

1. Physical Health:

- Quality sleep is a cornerstone of physical health. It allows the body to repair and regenerate tissues, maintain a strong immune system, and regulate essential functions like metabolism and hormone production.

2. Mental Health:

- Sleep plays a pivotal role in emotional regulation and cognitive function. Inadequate sleep is associated with mood disorders, increased stress, and reduced cognitive performance.

3. Productivity and Success:

- Prioritizing sleep enhances productivity, creativity, and decision-making, contributing to professional success and personal achievements.

4. Relationships:

- Healthy sleep habits can lead to improved interpersonal dynamics by reducing irritability, mood swings, and conflicts stemming from sleep deprivation.

5. Longevity:

- Chronic sleep deprivation is linked to an increased risk of chronic diseases and a shorter lifespan. Prioritizing sleep can promote a longer and healthier life.

6. Quality of Life:

- Adequate, restorative sleep contributes to an improved quality of life by fostering physical vitality, emotional well-being, and resilience to life's challenges.

Strategies for Prioritizing Sleep and Well-being

Recalling the insights from previous chapters, here are some strategies for making sleep a central component of your overall well-being:

1. Set Realistic Sleep Goals:

- Aim for 7-9 hours of quality sleep per night, aligning with your individual needs and lifestyle.

2. Create a Consistent Sleep Schedule:

- Go to bed and wake up at the same times each day, even on weekends, to regulate your body's internal clock.

3. Establish a Relaxing Bedtime Routine:

- Develop calming bedtime rituals that signal to your body that it's time to wind down.

4. Optimize Your Sleep Environment:

- Ensure your bedroom is conducive to sleep, with a comfortable mattress, darkness, and a cool temperature.

5. Mindful Technology Use:

- Reduce screen time before bed to avoid the disruptive effects of blue light on melatonin production.

6. Manage Stress and Anxiety:

- Practice stress-reduction techniques such as meditation, mindfulness, and deep breathing exercises.

7. Seek Professional Help:

- If you have persistent sleep problems or suspect a sleep disorder, consult a healthcare provider or sleep specialist for evaluation and treatment.

Creating a Personalized Sleep Plan

In this final chapter, we embark on the journey of creating a personalized sleep plan that aligns with your unique needs, preferences, and lifestyle. Understanding the importance of sleep, the factors that influence it, and the strategies for improvement is just the beginning. Now, it's time to take action and craft a plan that empowers you to achieve better sleep and, consequently, enhanced overall well-being.

Assessing Your Sleep Needs

Begin by assessing your individual sleep needs. Consider the following:

1. Ideal Sleep Duration:

- Reflect on how much sleep you need to feel your best. The recommended range is typically 7-9 hours for most adults, but individual variations exist.

2. Sleep Schedule:

- Determine your ideal bedtime and wake-up time. Consistency is key for regulating your internal body clock.

3. Sleep Environment:

- Evaluate your bedroom's comfort, darkness, noise levels, and temperature. Make adjustments to create an optimal sleep environment.

4. Sleep Quality:

- Reflect on the quality of your sleep. Do you often wake up feeling rested, or do you experience disturbances like frequent awakenings or vivid dreams?

Identifying Sleep Obstacles

Next, identify any obstacles or challenges that hinder your sleep. Common barriers may include:

1. Work Commitments:

- Are irregular work hours or excessive workload interfering with your ability to get enough sleep?

2. Lifestyle Factors:

- Are social engagements, excessive screen time, or a demanding social life affecting your sleep patterns?

3. Stress and Anxiety:

- Do stress and anxiety play a role in your sleep difficulties? Are there specific stressors you need to address?

4. Sleep Disorders:

- Have you noticed symptoms of sleep disorders, such as snoring, excessive daytime sleepiness, or restless legs?

Crafting Your Personalized Sleep Plan

Now, it's time to create your personalized sleep plan:

1. Set Realistic Goals:

- Based on your sleep needs and the barriers you've identified, set achievable sleep goals. These could include achieving a consistent sleep schedule, improving sleep quality, or addressing specific sleep disturbances.

2. Establish Healthy Sleep Habits:

- Implement evidence-based sleep hygiene practices, such as a calming bedtime routine, a comfortable sleep environment, and a mindful approach to technology use before bed.

3. Manage Stress and Anxiety:

- Incorporate stress-reduction techniques into your daily routine, such as meditation, yoga, or deep breathing exercises. Consider talking to a therapist or counselor if needed.

4. Seek Professional Help:

- If you suspect a sleep disorder or have persistent sleep problems, consult a healthcare provider or sleep specialist for evaluation and treatment options.

5. Monitor Your Progress:

- Keep a sleep diary to track your sleep patterns, habits, and progress toward your goals. Adjust your plan as needed based on your observations.

6. Prioritize Self-Care:

- Recognize that sleep is a form of self-care, and prioritize it as you would nutrition, exercise, and mental well-being.

Future Trends in Sleep Science and Health

As we conclude this exploration of sleep's vital role in our lives, let's take a glimpse into the future of sleep science and health. The field of sleep research is continually evolving, and new discoveries and technologies hold the promise of revolutionizing our understanding of sleep and its impact on well-being. In this final chapter, we'll discuss emerging trends and innovations that may shape the future of sleep science and health.

1. Personalized Sleep Medicine:

- Advancements in genetics and personalized medicine may enable tailored sleep interventions based on an individual's genetic makeup, lifestyle, and specific sleep patterns. This could lead to more effective treatments for sleep disorders.

2. Sleep Tracking Technology:

- Sleep tracking devices and apps are becoming increasingly sophisticated. Future innovations may provide more comprehensive and accurate data about sleep quality, including factors like sleep cycles, body temperature, and sleep-related movements.

3. Sleep and Mental Health Integration:

- A deeper understanding of the links between sleep and mental health is likely to result in more integrated approaches to treating mental health conditions. Sleep therapy may become a fundamental component of mental health care.

4. Sleep and Technology:

- While technology can disrupt sleep patterns, it also has the potential to assist in sleep improvement. We may see the development of smart sleep environments that optimize factors like lighting, temperature, and noise levels for restorative sleep.

5. Circadian Rhythm Management:

- Future research may yield more effective methods for managing circadian rhythms, which could benefit shift workers, travelers, and individuals with circadian rhythm disorders.

6. Sleep Education and Awareness:

- Increased recognition of the importance of sleep may lead to enhanced sleep education programs in schools and workplaces.

Promoting sleep as a vital component of overall health could become a cultural norm.

7. Sleep and Aging:

- As the aging population grows, there will be a greater focus on understanding age-related sleep issues and developing interventions to support healthy sleep in older adults.

8. Sleep as Preventive Medicine:

- Sleep may increasingly be recognized as a preventative measure against chronic diseases. Healthcare providers may prescribe sleep interventions alongside lifestyle changes to reduce the risk of conditions like diabetes and heart disease.

9. Ethical Considerations:

- As technologies like sleep tracking and enhancement become more sophisticated, ethical questions about data privacy, consent, and the potential for misuse may arise.

Don't miss out!

Visit the website below and you can sign up to receive emails whenever Gabriella Goldberger publishes a new book. There's no charge and no obligation.

https://books2read.com/r/B-A-CNJAB-KBWNC